Micronutrients Intake and Status during Pregnancy and Lactation

Micronutrients Intake and Status during Pregnancy and Lactation

Special Issue Editors

Louise Brough
Gail Rees

MDPI • Basel • Beijing • Wuhan • Barcelona • Belgrade

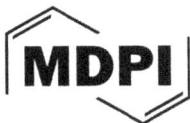

MDPI

Special Issue Editors
Louise Brough
Massey University
New Zealand

Gail Rees
University of Plymouth
UK

Editorial Office
MDPI
St. Alban-Anlage 66
4052 Basel, Switzerland

This is a reprint of articles from the Special Issue published online in the open access journal *Nutrients* (ISSN 2072-6643) from 2018 to 2019 (available at: https://www.mdpi.com/journal/nutrients/special_issues/Micronutrients_Pregnancy_Lactation)

For citation purposes, cite each article independently as indicated on the article page online and as indicated below:

LastName, A.A.; LastName, B.B.; LastName, C.C. Article Title. *Journal Name* **Year**, *Article Number*, Page Range.

ISBN 978-3-03897-840-4 (Pbk)
ISBN 978-3-03897–841-1 (PDF)

Contents

About the Special Issue Editors

Louise Brough is a Senior Lecturer in Human Nutrition at Massey University, Palmerston North, New Zealand. Her main research interest is micronutrient deficiency in pregnancy, lactation, and early life. She is currently focused on iodine, selenium, folate, and iron deficiency, both in developed and developing countries. She has research experience in the UK and New Zealand, and has collaborated on research endeavours focused in Africa. Dr Brough is currently a co-leader of the Massey Mother and Baby Nutrition Research Group

Gail Rees, PhD, is an Associate Professor in Human Nutrition at the University of Plymouth, UK. She is a registered nutritionist and dietitian. She has worked as a dietitian at the NHS for several years before taking a postdoctoral position at London Metropolitan University to work on a maternal micronutrient supplementation study in East London. A/Prof Rees currently teaches undergraduate and postgraduate nutritionists and dietitians, and leads the BSc (Hons) Nutrition Exercise and Health programme. Her research interests are in the field of maternal and child nutrition, and current research projects focus on obesity in pregnancy. She is also involved in the analysis of dietary data throughout childhood from the EarlyBird cohort study in Plymouth.

Preface to "Micronutrients Intake and Status during Pregnancy and Lactation"

Optimal nutrition is important during pregnancy and lactation for the health of both the mother and infant. Chronic deficiencies in both macronutrients and micronutrients are well recognised in developing countries. Although overconsumption of macronutrients is a major issue in developed countries, micronutrient deficiencies—which occur concomitantly—are no less of a concern. Furthermore, in developed countries, there is also the risk of excessive micronutrient intake from dietary supplements. Micronutrients have a role in foetal and neonatal health and, also, health in later life. Micronutrient deficiency or toxicity during pregnancy or early life can permanently affect developing tissues, resulting in adverse growth and development of the infant, which is associated with chronic diseases in adulthood. An aberrant micronutrient intake during pregnancy or lactation can also have a detrimental effect on the mother, both in the neonatal period and in later life. This book brings together some of the latest original research regarding micronutrients in pregnancy and lactation. Included are recent studies assessing the adequacy of the whole diet in both developing and developed countries. These studies consider a range of micronutrients consumed by pregnant and breastfeeding women. Other articles focus on micronutrients of particular concern among populations, such as iron, iodine, selenium, folate, and vitamin D, and investigate habitual intake, nutritional supplementation, and metabolism. The research presented in this book includes studies of pregnant and breastfeeding women at risk of nutritional deficiency and, also, micronutrient status and metabolism in women with obesity and gestational diabetes, and their effects on the neonate.

Louise Brough, Gail Rees
Special Issue Editors

nutrients

MDPI

Article

Use of Iodine-Containing Dietary Supplements Remains Low among Women of Reproductive Age in the United States: NHANES 2011–2014

Priya M. Gupta [1],*, Jaime J. Gahche [2], Kirsten A. Herrick [3], Abby G. Ershow [2], Nancy Potischman [2] and Cria G. Perrine [1]

[1]   Division of Nutrition, Physical Activity, and Obesity, Centers for Disease Control and Prevention, Atlanta, GA 30341, USA; cperrine@cdc.gov
[2]   National Institutes of Health, Office of Dietary Supplements, Bethesda, MD 20892, USA; jaime.gahche@nih.gov (J.J.G.); ershowa@od.nih.gov (A.G.E.); potischn@mail.nih.gov (N.P.)
[3]   National Center for Health Statistics, Centers for Disease Control and Prevention, Hyattsville, MD 20782, USA; kherrick1@cdc.gov
*   Correspondence: pmgupta@cdc.gov; Tel.:+1-908-418-0970

Received: 5 March 2018; Accepted: 27 March 2018; Published: 29 March 2018

check for updates

Abstract: In the United States, the American Thyroid Association recommends that women take a dietary supplement containing 150 µg of iodine 3 months prior to conception and while pregnant and lactating to support fetal growth and neurological development. We used data from the National Health and Nutrition Examination Survey 2011–2014 to describe the use of dietary supplements with and without iodine in the past 30 days among 2155 non-pregnant, non-lactating (NPNL) women; 122 pregnant women; and 61 lactating women. Among NPNL women, 45.3% (95% Confidence Interval [CI]: 42.0, 48.6) used any dietary supplement and 14.8% (95% CI: 12.7, 16.8) used a dietary supplement with iodine in the past 30 days. Non-Hispanic black and Hispanic women were less likely to use any dietary supplement as well as one with iodine, than non-Hispanic white or non-Hispanic Asian women ($p < 0.05$). Among pregnant women, 72.2% (95% CI: 65.8, 78.6) used any dietary supplement; however, only 17.8% (95% CI: 11.4, 24.3) used a dietary supplement with iodine. Among lactating women, 75.0% (95% CI: 63.0, 87.0) used a dietary supplement; however, only 19.0% (95% CI: 8.8, 29.2) used a dietary supplement with iodine. Among NPNL women using a supplement with iodine, median daily iodine intake was 75.0 µg. Self-reported data suggests that the use of iodine containing dietary supplements among pregnant and lactating women remains low in contrast with current recommendations.

Keywords: iodine; supplements; pregnant; lactating; women of reproductive age

1. Introduction

Iodine is an essential component of the thyroid hormones, thyroxine and triiodothyronine. These hormones regulate vital body functions including fetal and postnatal growth and neurologic development [1]. During pregnancy, iodine requirements increase to accommodate fetal needs and alterations in maternal iodine metabolism, including increased urinary iodine loss [2,3]. Adequate iodine intake is also critical early in pregnancy when the fetal brain is growing rapidly. Studies have shown that overt iodine deficiency is associated with irreversible neurological damage in the fetus [3]. Other studies suggest that even mild iodine deficiency is associated with poor cognitive development and educational attainment in young children [4,5].

The recommended daily allowance (RDA) of iodine for non-pregnant, non-lactating women (NPNL) is 150 µg/day and increases to 220 µg/day and 290 µg/day for pregnant and lactating women, respectively [6].

Given the increased demand for iodine during pregnancy and lactation, the high variability of iodine in foods [7–10] and the limited exposure to iodine from fortified salt [11], dietary intake alone may not be sufficient to ensure optimal iodine nutrition [8,12]. Therefore, it is important to monitor the use of dietary supplements containing iodine among women of reproductive age, as iodine is a nutrient critical for fetal brain development, and pregnant women in the US, as a group, may be iodine deficient [13].

In 2006, the American Thyroid Association (ATA) recommended that pregnant and lactating women in the United States and Canada take a dietary supplement containing 150 µg of iodine [14]. In 2014, the American Academy of Pediatrics (AAP) released a similar recommendation, advocating the use of an iodine supplement during pregnancy [15]. In 2017, the ATA added that women who are planning pregnancy should begin taking a supplement with iodine three months in advance of the planned pregnancy [16]. The last national estimates of iodine containing dietary supplement usage among women of reproductive age used data up to 2006 [17,18]. This study provides updated estimates of the prevalence of dietary supplement use (any or iodine-containing) among women of reproductive age (20–44 years, including pregnant and lactating women) in the United States.

2. Materials and Methods

2.1. Survey Design

The National Health and Nutrition Examination Survey (NHANES) is an ongoing, nationally representative survey of the civilian, non-institutionalized population in the United States. NHANES uses a complex, stratified, multistage probability cluster sampling design. Detailed information on the study design and methods is available elsewhere [19,20]. Briefly, data collection in NHANES includes a household interview and a physical examination conducted in the Mobile Examination Center (MEC). Informed consent was obtained from all adult participants, and the sampling protocol was approved by National Center for Health Statistics Research Ethics Review Board [20].

2.2. Sample Selection

To improve the reliability and stability of estimates, we pooled data from two cycles of NHANES: 2011–2012 and 2013–2014 (examination response rates for women were 69.4% and 68.8%, respectively) [21]. Pregnancy status was determined in the MEC. The MEC sample included 2517 women aged 20–44 years. Pregnancy status of adolescents (aged < 20 years) is not available in the publicly available NHANES data files; therefore, we limited our sample to adult women. Women were excluded if pregnancy status could not be ascertained (n = 179). The remaining 2338 women were further categorized into pregnant, lactating, and NPNL. Pregnant women were defined as those with a positive pregnancy test or self-reported pregnancy. Lactating women were those who reported that they were currently breastfeeding. NPNL women were defined as those who were not pregnant and did not report current breastfeeding. Two women were both pregnant and lactating; these women were included with the pregnant group only. Conceptually, we felt that pregnancy would drive supplement use more than lactation. We do not anticipate our results would change significantly, given there were only two women who were both pregnant and lactating. Our final analytic sample included 2338 women, of which 2155, 122, and 61 were NPNL, pregnant, and lactating, respectively.

2.3. Demographic Variables

Age was categorized into 5-year intervals: 20–24 years, 25–29 years, 30–34 years, 35–39 years, and 40–44 years. Self-reported race/Hispanic origin was categorized into: non-Hispanic white, non-Hispanic black, non-Hispanic Asian, and Hispanic. NHANES participants reporting 'other' race or multiple races are not shown separately, but are included in the overall and estimates for other demographic categorizations. Federal income to poverty ratio, calculated by dividing family income by the US Department of Health and Human Services poverty guidelines specific to the survey year, was categorized as follows: 0–185%, >185–350%, and >350% (based on WIC eligibility criteria) [22].

2.4. Dietary Supplement Data

Dietary supplement users included those who reported using any dietary supplement in the past 30 days, whereas iodine-containing supplement users were those that reported using a dietary supplement with iodine in the past 30 days. Data on dietary supplement use in the previous 30 days were collected during the household interview. Participants were asked about their usage of vitamins, minerals, herbals, and other dietary supplements; this included prescription and non-prescription products. Participants were then asked to show interviewers the containers for all products taken so that information from the label could be recorded, including product name and manufacturer or distributor name and address. Data were obtained from product labels post-interview for information on serving size, nutrients, and nutrient amounts. Participants were also asked about the frequency of use and amount typically used.

Descriptive statistics of daily iodine intake from supplements were derived among women who reported using a supplement with iodine (n = 323). The mean daily intakes of iodine reported in the NHANES total supplement files were pre-calculated by dividing the amount of iodine (based on the serving size listed on the product label) by the number of days the supplement had been used in the past 30 days. These methods are described in detail elsewhere [23,24]. Among iodine supplement users, frequency of iodine supplement use was categorized as 1–7, 8–15, 16–29, and 30 days.

2.5. Statistical Analyses

All statistical analyses were performed using SAS-Callable SUDAAN (version 11.0.1) software. MEC weights were used to account for NHANES's complex survey design (including oversampling) and survey non-response. Weighted prevalence estimates for use of at least one dietary supplement in the past 30 days and use of a dietary supplement containing iodine were calculated for all women. Prevalence estimates for all women and NPNL women were further stratified by age, race/Hispanic origin and family income to poverty ratio. Some sample sizes varied due to missing data on covariates, and this is indicated in table footnotes. Variance estimates for all statistics of interest were approximated by Taylor Series Linearization, accounting for the complex design of NHANES. Differences between groups were evaluated using a t statistic. Tests of linear trend across ordinal variables were evaluated using orthogonal contrast matrices. Statistical significance was set as $p < 0.05$. Estimates with a relative standard error ([(standard error of the prevalence/prevalence) * 100]) <30% are presented [25]. Stratified data for pregnant and lactating women are not presented due to small sample sizes. We did not account for multiple comparisons.

3. Results

3.1. All Women

Approximately half of women (47.6%; 95% CI: 44.3, 50.9) in our sample (including pregnant and lactating women) had used a dietary supplement in the past 30 days; however, 15.1% (95% CI: 13.2, 16.9) had used a dietary supplement containing iodine (Table 1). Younger women (aged 20–24 years) were significantly less likely to take any dietary supplements than women aged ≥25 years. Use of both any supplement and use of iodine-containing dietary supplements varied by race/Hispanic origin. For example, the prevalence of using any dietary supplement was significantly lower among non-Hispanic black women (35.3%; 95% CI: 30.6, 39.9) and Hispanic women (39.3%; 95% CI: 34.8, 43.9) compared to non-Hispanic white women (53.1%; 95% CI: 48.6, 57.5) and non-Hispanic Asian women (52.0%; 95% CI: 46.3, 57.7) women. In addition, the prevalence of using an iodine-containing dietary supplement was significantly lower among non-Hispanic black women (10.9%; 95% CI: 8.8, 13.1) as compared to non-Hispanic white women (17.1%; 95% CI: 14.0, 20.1) and non-Hispanic Asian women (14.4%; 95% CI: 11.8, 17.0) but did not significantly differ from that among Hispanic women (13.5%; 95% CI: 10.0, 17.0). Supplement use increased with income ($p < 0.05$ for linear trend). Women at or below 185% of the federal poverty level had a lower prevalence of any or iodine containing dietary supplement use as compared to women above 185% of the federal poverty level. A higher percentage of women with greater than a high school degree reported taking any supplement or iodine-containing dietary supplements than women with less than a high school degree.

Table 1. Prevalence of supplement use and iodine-containing supplement use among women of reproductive age (20–44 years) by demographic stratifications: NHANES 2011–2014.

	n	% Using Any Dietary Supplement [1]	95% Confidence Interval	% Using a Dietary Supplement with Iodine [1]	95% Confidence Interval
All women	2338	47.6	(44.3, 50.9)	15.1	(13.2, 16.9)
Age (years) [2]					
20–24	473	39.4 [a]	(32.6, 46.2)	10.9 [a]	(7.3, 14.5)
25–29	419	47.0 [b]	(40.9, 53.1)	16.1 [a,b]	(11.1, 21.1)
30–34	464	48.9 [b]	(43.0, 54.9)	16.2 [a,b]	(12.5, 19.9)
35–39	466	50.4 [b]	(43.5, 57.3)	14.4 [a,b]	(10.0, 18.8)
40–44	516	52.6 [b]	(46.9, 58.3)	18.0 [b]	(13.7, 22.3)
Race/Hispanic Origin [4]					
Non-Hispanic White	834	53.1 [a]	(48.6, 57.5)	17.1 [a]	(14.0, 20.1)
Non-Hispanic Black	533	35.3 [b]	(30.6, 39.9)	10.9 [b]	(8.8, 13.1)
Non-Hispanic Asian	343	52.0 [a]	(46.3, 57.7)	14.4 [a]	(11.8, 17.0)
All Hispanic	314	39.3 [b]	(34.8, 43.9)	13.5 [a,b]	(10.0, 17.0)
Poverty to Income Ratio [3,5]					
0–185%	1146	39.6 [a]	(35.0, 44.2)	9.9 [a]	(7.8, 12.1)
>185–350%	445	50.5 [b]	(43.8, 57.3)	16.9 [b]	(13.7, 20.0)
>350%	599	57.6 [b]	(51.7, 63.6)	20.4 [b]	(15.3, 25.5)
Education level [3,5]					
<High school degree	375	32.1 [a]	(27.4, 36.8)	8.3 [a]	(5.4, 11.2)
High school degree	411	42.6 [b]	(37.4, 47.8)	11.9 [a]	(8.4, 15.4)
>High school degree	1550	51.7 [c]	(47.5, 55.9)	17.1 [b]	(14.4, 19.8)
Non-pregnant, non-lactating women	2155	45.3	(42.0, 48.6)	14.8	(12.7, 16.8)
Age (years) [2]					
20–24	424	37.6 [a]	(30.1, 45.2)	11.1 [a]	(7.1, 15.2)
25–29	376	43.7 [a]	(37.2, 50.2)	16.6 [a,b]	(11.1, 22.1)
30–34	413	43.9 [a]	(38.4, 49.4)	14.8 [a,b]	(11, 18.7)
35–39	438	48.4 [a,b]	(41.2, 55.6)	13.3 [a,b]	(8.5, 18.0)
40–44	504	52.2 [b]	(46.4, 58.1)	18.2 [b]	(13.8, 22.6)
Race/Hispanic Origin [4]					
Non-Hispanic White	762	50.2 [a]	(45.5, 54.9)	16.6 [a]	(13.2, 19.9)
Non-Hispanic Black	489	34.7 [b]	(29.4, 40.0)	11.5 [b]	(9.3, 13.7)
Non-Hispanic Asian	317	50.2 [a]	(44.3, 56)	13.9 [a]	(11.0, 16.8)
All Hispanic	295	37.4 [b]	(32.9, 42)	13.2 [b]	(9.6, 16.6)
Poverty to Income Ratio [3,5]					
0–185%	1056	37.5 [a]	(32.9, 42.1)	10.1 [a]	(8.0, 12.2)
>185–350%	409	48.9 [b]	(42.1, 55.7)	16.3 [b]	(12.8, 19.9)
>350%	552	55.1 [b]	(48.6, 61.5)	20.2 [b]	(14.7, 25.7)
Education level [3,5]					
<High school degree	348	29.7 [a]	(24.6, 34.8)	8.7 [a]	(5.7, 11.8)
High school degree	384	41.4 [b]	(36.4, 46.4)	12.0 [a,b]	(8.3, 15.7)
>High school degree	1421	49.2 [c]	(45.1, 53.3)	16.7 [b]	(13.7, 19.6)
Pregnant women	122	72.2	(65.8, 78.6)	17.8	(11.4, 24.3)
Lactating women	61	75.0	(63.0, 87.0)	19.0	(8.8, 29.2)

[1] All analyses were weighted and took into account the complex survey design. Estimates that share the same superscript do not significantly differ from one another (significance is based on *t*-test values of $p < 0.05$). [2] Linear trend in any supplement use. [3] Linear trend in any supplement use and iodine-containing supplement use. [4] Other race/Hispanic origin is included in totals but not shown separately. [5] Sample sizes vary due to missing data.

3.2. Non-Pregnant, Non-Lactating Women

Less than half of NPNL women (45.3%; 95% CI: 42.0, 48.6) reported the use of a dietary supplement, and 14.8% (95% CI: 12.7, 16.8) reported the use of a dietary supplement containing iodine. A higher percentage of older women (aged 40–44 years) reported taking a dietary supplement (any or iodine-containing) as compared to younger women (aged 20–24 years) ($p < 0.05$). Non-Hispanic black and Hispanic women were significantly less likely to use a dietary supplement (any or iodine-containing) than non-Hispanic white or non-Hispanic Asian women. Prevalence estimates of dietary supplement use by federal income to poverty ratio and education level were similar to that of all women ($p < 0.05$ for linear trend for income and education level).

3.3. Pregnant Women

Although 72.2% (95% CI: 65.8, 78.6) of pregnant women reported using any dietary supplement, 17.8% (95% CI: 11.4, 24.3) reported using a dietary supplement with iodine.

3.4. Lactating Women

Among lactating women, 75.0% (95% CI: 63.0, 87.0) reported using a dietary supplement; however, 19.0% (95% CI: 8.8, 29.2) reported using a dietary supplement with iodine.

3.5. Daily Iodine Intake from Iodine-Containing Dietary Supplements

Among all women who reported using a dietary supplement with iodine, the daily intake of iodine from dietary supplements was right skewed. Median daily intake of iodine from dietary supplements was 75.0 µg among both all women and NPNL women (Table 2). Results for pregnant and lactating women are not shown due to small sample size.

Table 2. Daily intake of iodine from supplements containing iodine among women of reproductive age (20–44 years): NHANES 2011–2014 [1]

	n	Mean	95% Confidence Interval	Median	Interquartile Range
All women	323	88.3	(80.6, 96.1)	75.0	(113.0)
Non-pregnant, non-lactating women	295	87.8	(80.1, 95.5)	75.0	(114.0)

[1] Estimates of iodine intake are only among users of iodine-containing dietary supplements.

Half of all women who reported using a dietary supplement with iodine ($n = 323$) used the dietary supplement for the full 30 days. The percentages of women who reported using a dietary supplement with iodine for 1–7 days, 8–15 days, and 12–29 days were 15.1%, 18.6% and 16.4%, respectively (data not shown).

4. Discussion

About one in seven women of reproductive age (15.1%), including pregnant and lactating women, reported taking a dietary supplement that contained iodine. Two previous analyses of NHANES (1999–2006 and 2001–2006) described the prevalence of iodine-containing dietary supplement use among women of reproductive age [17,18]. At that time, approximately 20% of pregnant and non-pregnant women, and 15% of lactating women, were taking a dietary supplement that contained iodine. Our data suggest there has been little change since that time (17.8% pregnant and 19.0% lactating).

In 1999–2006, the median daily intake among women aged 15–39 years (including pregnant but not lactating) who reported taking a dietary supplement containing iodine was 124 µg/day [17]. This is higher than the 75 µg/day reported here, suggesting iodine intake among iodine supplement users may be lower than in previous years. While NHANES did oversample pregnant women in 1999–2006, the median iodine intake from supplements among NPNL women was 112 ug/day, compared to 75 ug/day for NPNL women in 2011–2014. This suggests that sample composition of the two study periods is not driving the difference in iodine intake from supplements.

It is important to note that both of these estimates are based on a 30-day frequency questionnaire. Therefore average daily nutrient intake over 30 days is calculated using information on the frequency of use, servings consumed, and iodine content in the serving (based on the product label); changes in median consumption can reflect changes in any of these three pieces of information. Our study found that 73.9% of women taking a supplement containing iodine were taking a product with at least 150 µg per serving (data not shown). Saldanha et al. found that for dietary supplements that were specifically marketed as prenatal supplements, the mean iodine content of prescription prenatal supplements was 150 ± 4.8 µg and for non-prescription prenatal supplements, it was 164 ± 6.7 ug [26]. As it is unlikely there has been a dramatic reduction in the amount of iodine included in dietary supplements containing at least some iodine, the lower median may be due to women reporting less frequent use of supplements. Data from the 1999–2006 NHANES indicated that 65% of women who reported using a dietary supplement with iodine used the supplement daily (unpublished data, Jaime Gahche, NIH). We found that only half of all women who reported using a dietary supplement with iodine used the dietary supplement daily, suggesting that frequency of iodine containing supplement use may be declining.

In 2014, the AAP released a recommendation for pregnant and lactating women to take a dietary supplement containing iodine [15], reinforcing the 2006 recommendation from ATA. While the majority of pregnant and lactating women in the current study were taking a supplement, our analysis suggests that many of the supplements consumed by these women do not contain iodine. An analysis in 2009 found that 51% of prenatal vitamins marketed in the US contained iodine [27], while a study published in 2017 found that 61% of commercially available prenatal vitamins in the US contained iodine [28]. Some of the increase in the inclusion of iodine in prenatal vitamins may be due to increased recognition by the supplement industry of the recommendations by various health agencies for iodine supplementation during pregnancy and lactation [28].

This study has several strengths. We used data from the NHANES, a nationally representative data source. We presented national estimates and estimates for various subsets of the US population, including the first nationally representative estimates for non-Hispanic Asian women. This study is also subject to limitations. First, the NHANES dietary supplement database relies on the manufacturers' labels to determine the amount of iodine in the products. The nutrient content of a dietary supplement can vary from what is reported on the nutrition label. A 2017 study by Andrews et al. found that the reported iodine content of a supplement can exceed the amount reported on the label by an average of 20.2% [29]. Second, we currently lack the appropriate database necessary for estimating the iodine intake from dietary sources; therefore, we are unable to estimate how much iodine supplements add to daily intakes. Currently, there is effort being taken in the US to develop a dietary database for iodine [30]. Third, we were limited by the small number of pregnant and lactating women. As a result, we were not able to produce estimates of the prevalence of dietary supplement use and iodine-containing dietary supplement use by sociodemographic characteristics among pregnant and lactating women.

In many countries, diet alone is not sufficient to meet the increased demand for iodine during pregnancy and lactation [8,12], and supplements may be an important source of additional iodine for these groups. Thus, it is necessary to monitor the use of dietary supplements containing iodine among key target groups.

Acknowledgments: The findings and conclusions in this report are those of the authors and do not necessarily represent the official position of the CDC or NIH.

Author Contributions: The authors' responsibilities were as follows—P.M.G., C.G.P., and J.J.G. had full access to all data in this study, were responsible for the integrity of the data and accuracy of the data analysis, and drafting the manuscript. P.M.G., C.G.P., K.A.H., A.G.E., N.P., and J.J.G. participated in the study design and interpretation of the data. C.G.P., K.A.H., A.G.E., N.P., and J.J.G. were responsible for critical revision of the manuscript. None of the authors had a financial or personal interest in any company or organization connected with the research represented in the article.

Conflicts of Interest: The authors declare no conflict of interest.

References

1. WHO/UNICEF/ICCIDD. *Assessment of Iodine Deficiency Disorders and Monitoring Their Elimination: A Guide for Program Managers*, 3rd ed.; World Health Organization: Geneva, Switzerland, 2001.
2. Glinoer, D. The regulation of thyroid function during normal pregnancy: Importance of the iodine nutrition status. *Best Pract. Res. Clin. Endocrinol. Metabol.* **2004**, *18*, 133–152. [CrossRef] [PubMed]
3. Zimmermann, M.B. Iodine deficiency in pregnancy and the effects of maternal iodine supplementation on the offspring: A review. *Am. J. Clin. Nutr.* **2009**, *89*, 668s–672s. [CrossRef] [PubMed]
4. Bath, S.C.; Steer, C.D.; Golding, J.; Emmett, P.; Rayman, M.P. Effect of inadequate iodine status in UK pregnant women on cognitive outcomes in their children: Results from the Avon Longitudinal Study of Parents and Children (ALSPAC). *Lancet* **2013**, *382*, 331–337. [CrossRef]
5. Hynes, K.L.; Otahal, P.; Hay, I.; Burgess, J.R. Mild iodine deficiency during pregnancy is associated with reduced educational outcomes in the offspring: 9-year follow-up of the gestational iodine cohort. *J. Clin. Endocrinol. Metab.* **2013**, *98*, 1954–1962. [CrossRef] [PubMed]
6. Institute of Medicine (US) Panel on Micronutrients. Dietary Reference Intakes for Vitamin A, Vitamin K, Arsenic, Boron, Chromium, Copper, Iodine, Iron, Manganese, Molybdenum, Nickel, Silicon, Vanadium, and Zinc. *J. Am. Diet Assoc.* **2001**, *101*, 294–301.
7. Bath, S.C.; Rayman, M.P. A review of the iodine status of UK pregnant women and its implications for the offspring. *Environ. Geochem. Health* **2015**, *37*, 619–629. [CrossRef] [PubMed]
8. Swanson, C.A.; Zimmermann, M.B.; Skeaff, S.; Pearce, E.N.; Dwyer, J.T.; Trumbo, P.R.; Zehaluk, C.; Andrews, K.W.; Carriquiry, A.; Caldwell, K.L.; et al. Summary of an NIH workshop to identify research needs to improve the monitoring of iodine status in the United States and to inform the DRI. *J. Nutr.* **2012**, *142*, 1175s–1185s. [CrossRef] [PubMed]
9. Zimmermann, M.B.; Andersson, M. Assessment of iodine nutrition in populations: Past, present, and future. *Nutr. Rev.* **2012**, *70*, 553–570. [CrossRef] [PubMed]
10. Dasgupta, P.K.; Liu, Y.; Dyke, J.V. Iodine Nutrition: Iodine Content of Iodized Salt in the United States. *Environ. Sci. Technol.* **2008**, *42*, 1315–1323. [CrossRef] [PubMed]
11. Quader, Z.S.; Patel, S.; Gillespie, C.; Cogswell, M.E.; Gunn, J.P.; Perrine, C.G.; Mattes, R.D.; Moshfegh, A. Trends and determinants of discretionary salt use: National Health and Nutrition Examination Survey 2003–2012. *Public Health Nutr.* **2016**, *19*, 2195–2203. [CrossRef] [PubMed]
12. Zimmermann, M.B.; Jooste, P.L.; Pandav, C.S. Iodine-deficiency disorders. *Lancet* **2008**, *372*, 1251–1262. [CrossRef]
13. Caldwell, K.L.; Makhmudov, A.; Ely, E.; Jones, R.L.; Wang, R.Y. Iodine status of the U.S. population, National Health and Nutrition Examination Survey, 2005–2006 and 2007–2008. *Thyroid* **2011**, *21*, 419–427. [CrossRef] [PubMed]
14. Becker, D.V.; Braverman, L.E.; Delange, F.; Dunn, J.T.; Franklyn, J.A.; Hollowell, J.G.; Lamm, S.H.; Mitchell, M.L.; Pearce, E.; Robbins, J.; et al. Iodine supplementation for pregnancy and lactation-United States and Canada: Recommendations of the American Thyroid Association. *Thyroid* **2006**, *16*, 949–951. [CrossRef] [PubMed]
15. American Academy of Pediatrics. Iodine Deficiency, Pollutant Chemicals, and the Thyroid: New Information on an Old Problem. *Pediatrics* **2014**, *133*, 1163–1166.
16. Alexander, E.K.; Pearce, E.N.; Brent, G.A.; Brown, R.S.; Chen, H.; Dosiou, C.; Grobman, W.A.; Laurberg, P.; Lazarus, J.H.; Mandel, S.J.; et al. 2017 Guidelines of the American Thyroid Association for the Diagnosis and Management of Thyroid Disease during Pregnancy and the Postpartum. *Thyroid* **2017**, *27*, 315–389. [CrossRef] [PubMed]
17. Gahche, J.J.; Bailey, R.L.; Mirel, L.B.; Dwyer, J.T. The prevalence of using iodine-containing supplements is low among reproductive-age women, NHANES 1999–2006. *J. Nutr.* **2013**, *143*, 872–877. [CrossRef] [PubMed]

18. Perrine, C.G.; Herrick, K.; Serdula, M.K.; Sullivan, K.M. Some subgroups of reproductive age women in the United States may be at risk for iodine deficiency. *J. Nutr.* **2010**, *140*, 1489–1494. [CrossRef] [PubMed]
19. National Center for Health Statistics. *National Center for Health Statistics. National Health and Nutrition Examination Survey: Analytic Guidelines, 2011–2012*; National Center for Health Statistics: Hyattsville, MD, USA, 2013.
20. National Center for Health Statistics. National Health and Nutrition Examination Survey: Sample Design, 2011–2014. Available online: https://wwwn.cdc.gov/nchs/nhanes/AnalyticGuidelines.aspx (accessed on 20 October 2017).
21. National Center for Health Statistics. NHANES Response Rates and Population Totals. Available online: https://www.cdc.gov/nchs/nhanes/response_rates_cps.htm (accessed on 20 October 2017).
22. U.S. Department of Health and Human Services. U.S. Federal Poverty Guidelines Used to Determine Financial Eligibility for Certain Federal Programs. Available online: https://aspe.hhs.gov/poverty-guidelines (accessed on 20 October 2017).
23. National Center for Health Statistics. National Health and Nutrition Examination Survey 2011–2012 Data Documentation, Codebook, and Frequencies Dietary Supplement Use 30-Day. Available online: https://wwwn.cdc.gov/Nchs/Nhanes/2011-2012/DSQTOT_G.htm (accessed on 20 October 2017).
24. National Center for Health Statistics. National Health and Nutrition Examination Survey 2013–2014 Data Documentation, Codebook, and Frequencies Dietary Supplement Use 30-Day. Available online: https://wwwn.cdc.gov/Nchs/Nhanes/2013-2014/DSQTOT_H.htm (accessed on 20 October 2017).
25. Centers for Disease Control and Prevention National Center for Health Statistics. *NHANES 1999–2000 Addendum to the NHANES III Analytic Guidelines*; National Center for Health Statistics: Atlanta, GA, USA, 2002.
26. Saldanha, L.G.; Dwyer, J.T.; Andrews, K.W.; Brown, L.L.; Costello, R.B.; Ershow, A.G.; Gusev, P.A.; Hardy, C.J.; Pehrsson, P.R. Is Nutrient Content and Other Label Information for Prescription Prenatal Supplements Different from Nonprescription Products? *J. Acad. Nutr. Diet.* **2017**, *117*, 1429–1436. [CrossRef] [PubMed]
27. Leung, A.M.; Pearce, E.N.; Braverman, L.E. Iodine Content of Prenatal Multivitamins in the United States. *N. Engl. J. Med.* **2009**, *360*, 939–940. [CrossRef] [PubMed]
28. Lee, S.Y.; Stagnaro-Green, A.; MacKay, D.; Wong, A.W.; Pearce, E.N. Iodine Contents in Prenatal Vitamins in the United States. *Thyroid* **2017**, *27*, 1101–1102. [CrossRef] [PubMed]
29. Andrews, K.W.; Gusev, P.A.; Dang, P.; Savarala, S.; Oh, L.; Atkinson, R.; McNeal, M. Adult Multivitamin/mineral (AMVM-2017) Dietary Supplement Study Research Summary. Available online: https://dietarysupplementdatabase.usda.nih.gov/dsid_database/Res%20Summ%20DSID%204%20Adult%20MVM-8-2-17%20final.pdf (accessed on 5 January 2018).
30. Ershow, A.G.; Skeaff, S.A.; Merkel, J.M.; Pehrsson, P.R. Development of Databases on Iodine in Foods and Dietary Supplements. *Nutrients* **2018**, *10*, 100.

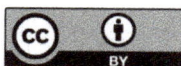

nutrients

MDPI

Article

Trimester-Specific Dietary Intakes in a Sample of French-Canadian Pregnant Women in Comparison with National Nutritional Guidelines

Claudia Savard [1,2,3], Simone Lemieux [1,3], S. John Weisnagel [2,4], Bénédicte Fontaine-Bisson [5,6], Claudia Gagnon [2,3,4], Julie Robitaille [1,2,3] and Anne-Sophie Morisset [1,2,3,*]

[1] School of Nutrition, Laval University, Québec City, QC G1V 0A6, Canada; claudia.savard.4@ulaval.ca (C.S.); simone.lemieux@fsaa.ulaval.ca (S.L.); julie.robitaille@fsaa.ulaval.ca (J.R.)
[2] Endocrinology and Nephrology Unit, CHU de Québec-Université Laval Research Center, Québec City, QC G1V 4G2, Canada; john.weisnagel@crchudequebec.ulaval.ca (S.J.W.); claudia.gagnon@crchudequebec.ulaval.ca (C.G.)
[3] Institute of Nutrition and Functional Foods, Laval University, Québec City, QC G1V 0A6, Canada
[4] Department of Medicine, Laval University, Québec City, QC G1V 0A6, Canada
[5] School of Nutrition Sciences, University of Ottawa, Ottawa, ON K1N 6N5, Canada; bfontain@uottawa.ca
[6] Institut du Savoir Montfort, Montfort Hospital, Ottawa, ON K1K 0T2, Canada
* Correspondence: anne-sophie.morisset@fsaa.ulaval.ca; Tel.: +1-418-656-2131 (ext. 13982)

check for updates

Received: 14 May 2018; Accepted: 12 June 2018; Published: 14 June 2018

Abstract: Diet during pregnancy greatly impacts health outcomes. This study aims to measure changes in dietary intakes throughout trimesters and to assess pregnant women's dietary intakes in comparison with current Canadian nutritional recommendations. Seventy-nine pregnant women were recruited and completed, within each trimester, three Web-based 24-h dietary recalls and one Web questionnaire on supplement use. Dietary intakes from food, with and without supplements, were compared to nutritional recommendations throughout pregnancy. Energy and macronutrient intakes remained stable throughout pregnancy. A majority of women exceeded their energy and protein requirements in the first trimester, and fat intakes as a percentage of energy intakes were above recommendations for more than half of the women in all trimesters. Supplement use increased dietary intakes of most vitamins and minerals, but 20% of women still had inadequate total vitamin D intakes and most women had excessive folic acid intakes. This study showed that pregnant women did not increase their energy intakes throughout pregnancy as recommended. Furthermore, although prenatal supplementation reduces the risk of inadequate intake for most micronutrients, there is still a risk of excessive folic acid and insufficient vitamin D intake, which needs further investigation.

Keywords: pregnancy; dietary intakes; energy intakes; supplements; dietary reference intakes (DRIs)

1. Introduction

Pregnancy is a critical period during which the pregnant woman's diet must provide enough nutrients to ensure optimal fetal development as well as to sustain the mother's physiological needs. In fact, in addition to the metabolic demand associated with the fetus' growth, rises in blood volume, extracellular liquids, adipose tissue, and placental weight all lead to an increase in the mother's dietary requirements [1,2]. Consequently, as recommended by the Institute of Medicine and Health Canada, daily pre-pregnancy energy intakes should be increased by 340 and 452 kcal in the second and third trimesters, respectively, in order to create a positive energy balance [3,4]. Likewise, pregnant women should increase their protein intakes in the second and third trimesters, but no specific recommendation exists for carbohydrates and fats during pregnancy [3].

Higher energy intakes should allow pregnant women to meet their higher essential fatty acid, dietary fiber, folic acid, iron, vitamin D, calcium, vitamin B_{12}, and vitamin C requirements [3,4]. However, previous research highlighted various dietary inadequacies, namely folate, iron, vitamin B_{12}, and vitamin D insufficiencies [5–7] thus suggesting that pregnant women may have difficulty meeting their higher micronutrient requirements through diet alone [5]. Moreover, since inadequate folate and iron status during pregnancy has been associated with numerous adverse health outcomes [8–10], Health Canada recommends that pregnant women should take, on a daily basis, a multivitamin that contains at least 400 µg of folic acid and 16–20 mg of iron [4]. There are currently no specific recommendations in terms of supplementation for other micronutrients. The use of a multivitamin combined with the increase in total energy intakes is probably sufficient to allow pregnant women to fill other micronutrient requirements [11].

Dietary intakes should be examined throughout pregnancy in order to detect potential excesses or deficiencies in macro- and micronutrients associated with adverse pregnancy outcomes [12–14]. However, to date, few studies have assessed pregnant women's dietary intakes by considering both food and supplement sources, and even fewer have done so in each trimester of pregnancy [15–20]. To our knowledge, no study assessed trimester-specific adequacy to current nutritional Canadian recommendations. This study aimed to: (1) measure changes in energy and macronutrient intakes across trimesters; and (2) assess pregnant women's dietary intakes in comparison with current Canadian nutritional recommendations.

2. Materials and Methods

2.1. Study Population

Eighty-six (86) pregnant women recruited from April 2016 to May 2017 at the CHU de Québec—Université Laval (Québec City, QC, Canada) were included in the ANGE (*Apports Nutritionnels durant la GrossessE*) project. Women younger than 18 years old and with a gestational age greater than 11 weeks of pregnancy at the time of recruitment were excluded. Women with a previously diagnosed severe medical condition (i.e., type 1 or type 2 diabetes, renal disease, inflammatory and autoimmune disorders) were also excluded. Our final sample included 79 women for whom we have nutritional data in all trimesters. The ANGE project was approved by the CHU de Québec—Université Laval Research Center's Ethics Committee and participants gave their informed written consent at their first visit to the research center.

2.2. The Automated Web-Based 24-h Recall (R24W)

In the first (range: 8.4–14.0 weeks), second (range: 19.3–28.3 weeks), and third (range: 31.9–37.7 weeks) trimesters of pregnancy, each participant was asked to complete a total of three Web-based 24-h dietary recalls, using the R24W (Rappel de 24h Web; 24h dietary recall) platform, on two weekdays and one weekend day (total of nine dietary recalls throughout pregnancy). The development of the R24W has been previously described [21]. Briefly, the R24W uses a sequence of questions inspired by the United States Department of Agriculture (USDA) Automated Multiple Pass Method (AMPM) [22]. The application sends automatic emails on randomly chosen dates to remind the participants to complete the recall. Participants were required to watch a mandatory tutorial video prior to their first recall. The database includes 2865 food items that are linked to the Canadian Nutrient File [23] to enable automatic extraction of nutrient values. Participants can report an unlimited number of meals and snacks for a 24-h period. Pictures depicting multiple portion sizes with corresponding units and/or volume are available for more than 80% of all food items. After selecting a food item, participants must choose the picture that best represents the amount of food eaten. In addition, systematic questions are asked about frequently forgotten food items including toppings, condiments, fats, snacks, and drinks. The R24W was previously validated in pregnant women for each trimester [24]. All food items were automatically coded using the 2015 version of the Canadian Nutrient File [23] and data for energy and 22 nutrients were analyzed.

2.3. Supplement Use

Information regarding dietary and prenatal supplement use was obtained through a Web questionnaire administered within each trimester. Participants had to identify their supplement (e.g., brand name, type of supplement, specific nutrient, etc.), and provide its drug identification number (DIN), its measurement unit (e.g., tablets, drops, grams, milliliters, etc.), the dosage, and the frequency at which the reported dose was taken. Participants could enter as many as 10 dietary supplements. The Health Canada Licensed Natural Health Product Database [25] as well as companies' product labels and websites were used to collect the nutritional information of all supplements entered by participants. If information was missing or was incomplete for any of the supplements' characteristics, a research assistant contacted the participant to obtain the missing information. We assessed supplement use by compiling types of supplements used (multivitamins or single-nutrient supplements) and the number of users for each type of supplement.

2.4. Estimated Energy and Protein Requirements

Pre-pregnancy body weight was self-reported and height was measured at baseline to calculate pre-pregnancy BMI. Participants completed the validated French version of the Pregnancy Physical Activity Questionnaire (PPAQ) [26,27] within each trimester. Physical activity levels (PALs) were determined by ranking the participants according to the total amount of time they engaged in moderate and high-intensity activities (minutes/day). According to the Institute of Medicine (IOM) guidelines for the general adult population (which includes pregnant women) [3], participants were either considered sedentary (less than 30 min of moderate-intensity activity), low-active (30 to 60 min of moderate-intensity activity), active (60 to 180 min of moderate-intensity activity or 30 to 60 min of high-intensity activity) or very active (more than 180 min of moderate-intensity activity or more than 60 min of high-intensity activity). Estimated energy requirements (EERs) were calculated for each trimester by using pre-pregnancy weight, age, height, and physical activity coefficient corresponding to the PAL determined by the PPAQ [3]. An additional 340 kcal and 452 kcal were respectively added to the second and third trimester EERs [3]. Daily protein requirements were calculated as 1.1 g/kg of pre-pregnancy weight for the first 20 weeks of pregnancy, to which 25 g of protein per day was added for the remaining 20 weeks of pregnancy [3].

2.5. Other Variables

Gestational age (weeks of gestation) was confirmed by ultrasound conducted at the CHU de Québec—Université Laval in the first trimester. A Web-based self-administered questionnaire was completed by all participants either in the first ($n = 62$) or in the second ($n = 24$) trimester to collect information on economic and socio-demographic characteristics.

2.6. Statistical Analyses

within each trimester, means and standard deviations for energy and macro- and micronutrient intakes as well as the percentage of energy from carbohydrates (% carbohydrates), fat (% fat), and proteins (% proteins) were calculated from the three 24-h dietary recalls. Total micronutrient intakes were calculated by combining intakes from supplements and intakes from food sources only (derived from the dietary recalls). We then compared total energy and nutrient intakes and intakes from food sources only with dietary reference intakes (DRIs) by calculating proportions of women that had intakes below the estimated average intakes (EARs) and above the upper intake limit (UL), as applicable [28]. Folate intakes as dietary folate equivalent (DFE) were compared to the EAR (520 µg), and only synthetic forms of folic acid (i.e., fortified foods and supplements) were compared to the UL for folic acid (1000 µg), as the UL for folic acid applies only to synthetic forms [3]. Similarly, only niacin and magnesium intakes from supplements were compared to the UL for these nutrients, as their respective UL only applies to intakes from supplements [3]. Energy intakes (EIs) were compared with EERs, and protein, carbohydrate, and fat intakes as percentages of energy were compared with the acceptable macronutrient distribution range (AMDR) [3]. Proportions of women with values below or above the EERs or AMDR were calculated. Protein intakes (g/day) were also compared to estimated protein requirements, as previously described [3]. Finally, repeated measures ANOVA was performed to assess variations in energy, macro- and micronutrient intakes across trimesters. All statistical analyses were performed in JMP version 13 (SAS Institute Inc., Cary, NC, USA).

3. Results

Participant characteristics are presented in Table 1. Of the 86 pregnant women recruited, seven were lost to follow-up, mainly due to miscarriage or lack of time to devote to the project. Therefore, results include 79 pregnant women with a mean age of 32.1 ± 3.7 years and an average pre-pregnancy BMI of 25.7 ± 5.8 kg/m^2. The majority of participants were Caucasian (97.5%), had a university degree (78.5%), an annual household income of C\$80,000 or more (63.3%), and were multiparous (64.6%).

Table 1. Participants' characteristics (*n* = 79).

Variables	Mean ± SD or *N* (%)
Age (years)	32.1 ± 3.7
Weeks of gestation at baseline (weeks)	9.3 ± 0.7
Primiparous	28 (35.4)
BMI (kg/m^2)	25.7 ± 5.8
Underweight	2 (2.5)
Normal weight	43 (54.4)
Overweight	19 (24.1)
Obese	15 (19.0)
Ethnicity–Caucasian	77 (97.5)
Education	
High school	4 (5.0)
College	13 (16.5)
University	62 (78.5)
Household income	
<C\$40,000	5 (6.3)
C\$40,000–59,999	10 (12.7)
C\$60,000–79,999	13 (16.5)
C\$80,000–99,999	17 (21.5)
>C\$100,000	33 (41.8)
Income missing	1 (1.2)
Physical activity level (minutes of moderate and vigorous activity/day)	
First trimester	60.5 ± 59.6
Second trimester	45.9 ± 51.1
Third trimester	35.2 ± 41.5

3.1. Supplement Use

Prenatal multivitamins were used by a majority of pregnant women (86.1%, 84.8%, and 78.5% in the first, second, and third trimesters, respectively) and folic acid supplements were the most commonly reported single-nutrient supplements (data not shown). Among women that did not take a multivitamin, the most reported single nutrient taken was folic acid for all trimesters (data not shown). Furthermore, among participants taking two supplements, the most reported single nutrients combined with a multivitamin were folic acid (50.0%) vitamin D (40.0%), and iron (44.4%) in the first, second, and third trimesters, respectively (data not shown). Small proportions (<10%) of women reported taking vitamin D, iron, and omega-3 as single-nutrient supplements throughout pregnancy (data not shown). In the third trimester, women who reported taking no supplement were significantly younger than the women who were taking at least one supplement (30.3 $\pm$ 3.8 years old vs. 32.6 $\pm$ 3.5 years old, p = 0.0236; data not shown).

3.2. Energy, Macronutrients, and Dietary Fiber

Table 2 shows trimester-specific energy intakes and macronutrient intakes as percentages of energy intake derived from the dietary recalls in comparison with EERs and AMDRs. No significant difference was observed for energy, protein, carbohydrate, or lipid intakes across trimesters. However, a significant increase in SFAs and a decrease in PUFAs as percentages of energy intakes were observed across trimesters (Table 2). Macronutrient intakes (grams per day) derived from the R24Ws and proportions of women that reported intakes above or below the corresponding DRIs are shown in Table 3. Mean energy intakes exceeded EERs in the first trimester (2294.3 $\pm$ 487.2 vs. 2122.4 $\pm$ 265.9 kcal; p = 0.006), but were below EERs in the third trimester (2234.6 $\pm$ 476.1 vs. 2492.2 $\pm$ 216.8 kcal; p < 0.0001). Protein intakes as a percentage of energy were within the acceptable distribution range (10–35%) in all trimesters but exceeded estimated requirements (1.1 g/kg) in the first trimester (96.7 $\pm$ 20.7 vs. 70.0 $\pm$ 8.6 g/day; p < 0.0001) for almost all participants (94.9% of them). In all trimesters, a majority of women reported fat intakes that were above the acceptable distribution range as a percentage of energy intakes. Inversely, carbohydrate intakes as percentages of energy were below the acceptable distribution range for more than 20% of participants for each trimester. Dietary fiber intakes were also below the DRI of 14 g/1000 kcal in all trimesters for more than 85% of participants.

3.3. Vitamins and Minerals

Micronutrient intakes derived from the R24Ws (food sources only) and proportions of women that reported intakes above or below the corresponding DRIs are shown in Table 4. A high prevalence of inadequate intakes was observed for vitamin D (93.7%, 83.5%, 78.5%), iron (88.6%, 89.9%, 94.9%), and folate (58.2%, 60.8%, 68.4%) in all trimesters, when only food sources were considered (Table 4). Vitamin B_6 intakes were below the EAR for 36.7%, 32.9%, and 38.0% of women in the first, second, and third trimesters, respectively. Smaller proportions of women reported, throughout pregnancy, inadequate intakes of magnesium, vitamin A, calcium, and zinc. Vitamin C intakes were inadequate for 22.8% of participants in the second trimester but only for 4.1% and 10.1% of women in the first and third trimesters, respectively. Repeated measures ANOVA showed significant decreases in dietary intakes of vitamin C and manganese, as well as significant increases in dietary calcium and vitamin B_{12} intakes across trimesters (Table 4). In all trimesters, a majority of pregnant women reported sodium intakes that were above the UL of 2300 mg.

As shown in Table 5, when food sources and dietary supplements were combined, the proportion of women with adequate micronutrient intakes increased. With the exception of folate, vitamin D, and iron, less than 15% of our participants had total micronutrient intakes below the EAR, in all trimesters. Total intakes of folic acid and sodium were above the UL for a majority of women, and more than a third of participants had total iron intakes above the UL for all trimesters. The significant decrease observed for vitamin C and manganese, as well as the significant increase in calcium intakes persisted after the addition of intakes from supplements (Table 5).

Table 2. Trimester-specific energy intakes and macronutrient intakes as percentage of energy intakes in comparison with dietary reference intakes.

	First Trimester			Second Trimester			Third Trimester			p-Value [a]
	Mean ± SD or AMDR Range	%Below AMDR or EER	%Above AMDR or EER	Mean ± SD or AMDR Range	%Below AMDR or EER	%Above AMDR or EER	Mean ± SD or AMDR Range	%Below AMDR or EER	%Above AMDR or EER	
EER (kcal/day)	2122.4 ± 265.9	-	-	2403.4 ± 241.1	-	-	2492.2 ± 216.8	-	-	-
Energy intake (kcal/day)	2294.3 ± 487.2	36.7	63.3	2320.2 ± 519.1	60.8	39.2	2234.6 ± 476.1	70.9	29.1	0.09
AMDR protein, E%	10–35	-	-	10–35	-	-	10–35	-	-	-
Protein, E%	16.9 ± 2.5	0	0	17.3 ± 2.9	0	0	17.9 ± 3.3	0	0	0.14
AMDR carbohydrate, E%	45–65	-	-	45–65	-	-	45–65	-	-	-
Carbohydrate, E%	49.4 ± 4.7	20.3	0	48.3 ± 5.7	24.1	0	48.3 ± 5.5	24.1	0	0.27
AMDR total fat, E%	20–35	-	-	20–35	-	-	20–35	-	-	-
Total fat, E%	35.1 ± 4.0	0	50.6	35.8 ± 4.9	0	55.7	35.5 ± 4.4	0	57.0	0.53
SFA, E%	12.8 ± 2.1	-	-	13.2 ± 2.9	-	-	13.5 ± 2.5	-	-	0.047
MUFA, E%	12.3 ± 2.1	-	-	12.6 ± 2.0	-	-	12.5 ± 2.1	-	-	0.49
PUFA, E%	7.1 ± 1.9	-	-	7.1 ± 2.0	-	-	6.5 ± 1.8	-	-	0.03

[a] *p*-value for repeated measures ANOVA performed to assess variations in energy and macronutrient intakes across trimesters. When no dietary reference intake was established for a nutrient, the "-" is used instead of a 0. AMDR: acceptable macronutrient distribution range; EER: estimated energy requirement, calculated with the following formula: 354 − (6.91 × age) + physical activity coefficient × [(9.36 × weight) + (726 × height)], to which an additional 340 or 452 kcal were added in the second and third trimesters. SFA: saturated fatty acids; MUFA: monounsaturated fatty acids; PUFA: polyunsaturated fatty acids.

Table 3. Trimester-specific macronutrient intakes in comparison with dietary reference intakes.

	First Trimester			Second Trimester			Third Trimester			p-Value [a]
	Mean ± SD	%Below EPR or AI	%Above EPR or AI	Mean ± SD	%Below EPR or AI	%Above EPR or AI	Mean ± SD	%Below EPR or AI	%Above EPR or AI	
EPR, g/day	70.0 ± 8.6	-	-	95.0 ± 8.6	-	-	95.0 ± 8.6	-	-	-
Protein, g/day	96.7 ± 20.7	5.1	94.9	99.1 ± 20.9	48.1	51.9	98.2 ± 22.0	43.0	57.0	0.64
Carbohydrate, g/day	283.3 ± 68.8	-	-	280.3 ± 70.9	-	-	270.1 ± 68.0	-	-	0.14
Total fat, g/day	89.6 ± 21.7	-	-	93.1 ± 27.5	-	-	88.6 ± 23.6	-	-	0.20
Dietary fiber, g/day	23.3 ± 7.0	96.2	3.8	23.9 ± 8.0	87.3	12.7	22.9 ± 6.7	89.9	10.1	0.50
ω-6 Linoleic acid, g/day	14.8 ± 5.4	-	-	14.5 ± 5.3	-	-	13.4 ± 5.3	-	-	0.07
ω-3 Linolenic acid, g/day	2.0 ± 0.7	-	-	2.0 ± 0.9	-	-	1.9 ± 0.9	-	-	0.38
Cholesterol, mg/day	297.2 ± 99.7	-	-	291.1 ± 91.7	-	-	288.1 ± 109.0	-	-	0.81

[a] *p*-value for repeated measures ANOVA performed to assess variations in macronutrient intakes across trimesters. When no dietary reference intake was established for a nutrient, the "-" is used instead of a 0. EPR: estimated protein requirement (1.1 g/kg or pre-pregnancy weight for the first half of pregnancy and 1.1 g/kg of pre-pregnancy weight + 25 g for the second half). AI: adequate intake.

Table 4. Trimester-specific micronutrient intakes from food alone in comparison with dietary reference intakes.

	EAR	UL	First Trimester			Second Trimester			Third Trimester			p-Value [a]
			Mean ± SD	%Below EAR	%Above UL	Mean ± SD	%Below EAR	%Above UL	Mean ± SD	%Below EAR	%Above UL	
Vitamin D, IU/day	400	4000	234.8 ± 119.0	93.7	0	261.2 ± 135.2	83.5	0	271.9 ± 150.2	78.5	0	0.11
Iron, mg/day	22	45	15.3 ± 4.8	88.6	0	15.8 ± 5.2	89.9	0	14.8 ± 4.2	94.9	0	0.09
Folate, µg DFE/day	520	-	516.2 ± 139.5	58.2	-	495.4 ± 143.3	60.8	-	490.1 ± 141.3	68.4	-	0.31
Folic acid, µg/day	-	1000	155.0 ± 65.5	-	0	146.8 ± 72.6	-	0	138.3 ± 72.1	-	0	0.17
Vitamin B_6, mg/day	1.6	100	1.8 ± 0.5	36.7	0	1.9 ± 0.5	32.9	0	1.8 ± 0.5	38.0	0	0.32
Magnesium, mg/day	290–300	350	381.2 ± 103.8	17.8	-	391.9 ± 108.9	19.0	-	386.2 ± 106.4	20.3	-	0.65
Vitamin A, µg RAE/day	550	3000	879.2 ± 305.9	13.9	0	906.4 ± 392.5	17.7	0	916.2 ± 398.4	17.7	0	0.71
Zinc, mg/day	9.5	40	12.5 ± 3.2	12.7	0	13.4 ± 3.2	8.9	0	13.2 ± 3.7	11.4	0	0.15
Calcium, mg/day	800	2500	1292.3 ± 381.8	10.1	0	1350.3 ± 515.9	13.9	2.5	1427.0 ± 506.0	6.3	1.3	0.02
Vitamin C, mg/day	70	2000	159.5 ± 66.7	5.1	0	137.9 ± 81.4	22.8	0	138.4 ± 66.6	10.1	0	0.01
Thiamin, mg/day	1.2	-	1.9 ± 0.6	5.1	-	1.9 ± 0.7	7.6	-	1.8 ± 0.8	7.6	-	0.40
Vitamin B_{12}, µg/day	2.2	-	4.8 ± 1.6	2.5	-	5.4 ± 2.4	3.8	-	5.6 ± 2.5	0	-	0.02
Riboflavin, mg/day	1.2	-	2.3 ± 0.6	1.3	-	2.4 ± 0.6	1.3	-	2.5 ± 0.8	0	-	0.07
Niacin, mg NE/day	14	35	45.7 ± 10.6	0	-	45.9 ± 9.2	0	-	45.0 ± 10.3	0	-	0.64
Pantothenic acid, mg/day	-	-	6.5 ± 1.8	-	-	6.5 ± 1.5	-	-	6.5 ± 1.6	-	-	0.98
Phosphorus, mg/day	580	3500	1616.4 ± 383.7	0	0	1660.3 ± 398.0	0	0	1673.7 ± 442.1	0	0	0.47
Sodium, mg/day	-	2300	3406.0 ± 889.8	-	94.9	3276.0 ± 950.3	-	86.1	3199.0 ± 921.7	-	84.8	0.17
Manganese, mg/day	-	11	4.0 ± 1.5	-	1.3	4.3 ± 1.4	-	-	3.9 ± 1.3	-	-	0.005
Selenium, µg/day	49	400	135.7 ± 34.0	0	0	135.2 ± 32.1	0	0	131.8 ± 30.9	0	0	0.48
Copper, mg/day	0.8	10	1.5 ± 0.6	1.3	0	1.6 ± 0.6	1.3	0	1.5 ± 0.5	3.8	0	0.22

[a] *p*-value for repeated measures ANOVA performed to assess variations in micronutrient intakes across trimesters. When no EAR or UL was established for a nutrient, the "-" is used instead of a 0. EAR: estimated average requirement; UL: upper intake limit; DFE: dietary folate equivalent; RAE: retinol activity equivalents; NE: niacin equivalent.

Table 5. Trimester-specific total micronutrient intakes (including food sources and supplements) in comparison with dietary reference intakes.

	EAR	UL	First Trimester			Second Trimester			Third Trimester			p-Value [a]
			Mean ± SD	%Below EAR	%Above UL	Mean ± SD	%Below EAR	%Above UL	Mean ± SD	%Below EAR	%Above UL	
Vitamin D, IU/day	400	4000	632.2 ± 555.9	25.3	1.3	690.0 ± 538.4	21.5	1.3	689.4 ± 544.9	21.5	1.3	0.15
Iron, mg/day	22	45	38.2 ± 14.0	19.0	35.4	38.8 ± 13.8	19.0	38.0	41.0 ± 24.7	22.8	36.7	0.65
Folate, µg DFE/day	520	-	1777.0 ± 1221.4	7.6	-	1763.2 ± 1313.0	10.1	-	1617.6 ± 1212.2	16.5	-	0.29
Folic acid, µg/day	-	1000	1415.8 ± 1213.7	-	86.1	1412.6 ± 1313.4	-	83.5	1265.8 ± 1199.3	-	79.7	0.27
Vitamin B$_6$, mg/day	1.6	100	5.6 ± 3.9	8.9	0	5.8 ± 4.0	7.6	0	5.4 ± 4.0	8.9	0	0.29
Magnesium, mg/day	290–300	350	419.1 ± 108.4	8.9	0	431.9 ± 113.9	8.9	0	424.2 ± 110.8	11.4	0	0.62
Vitamin A, µg RAE/day	550	3000	1398.1 ± 574.4	7.6	0	1415.9 ± 674.8	7.6	0	1429.8 ± 635.5	7.6	0	0.91
Zinc, mg/day	9.5	40	20.4 ± 6.7	5.1	0	21.4 ± 6.6	2.5	0	21.0 ± 7.2	3.8	0	0.36
Calcium, mg/day	800	2500	1503.4 ± 370.6	2.5	0	1560.0 ± 551.4	6.3	5.1	1630.7 ± 524.4	2.5	6.3	0.04
Vitamin C, mg/day	70	2000	234.7 ± 79.1	1.3	0	215.7 ± 93.3	7.6	0	213.2 ± 71.0	2.5	0	0.04
Thiamin, mg/day	1.2	-	3.4 ± 1.3	2.5	-	3.5 ± 1.3	2.5	-	3.3 ± 1.4	2.5	-	0.31
Vitamin B$_{12}$, µg/day	2.2	-	11.0 ± 8.0	1.3	-	10.6 ± 5.7	0	-	10.1 ± 5.3	0	-	0.54
Riboflavin, mg/day	1.2	-	4.0 ± 1.4	1.3	-	4.1 ± 1.5	0	-	4.1 ± 1.5	0	-	0.80
Niacin, mg NE/day	14	35	60.1 ± 13.4	0	-	60.8 ± 12.8	0	-	59.3 ± 14.6	0	-	0.64
Pantothenic acid, mg/day	-	-	11.1 ± 3.2	-	-	11.1 ± 3.1	-	-	10.9 ± 3.1	-	-	0.86
Phosphorus, mg/day	580	3500	1618.0 ± 383.6	0	0	1665.7 ± 401.2	0	0	1673.7 ± 442.1	0	0	0.49
Sodium, mg/day	-	2300	3406.0 ± 889.8	-	94.9	3276.0 ± 950.3	-	86.1	3199.0 ± 921.7	-	84.8	0.17
Manganese, mg/day	-	11	5.0 ± 1.9	-	1.3	5.3 ± 1.8	-	1.3	4.9 ± 1.6	-	1.3	0.04
Selenium, µg/day	49	400	151.2 ± 38.1	0	0	151.4 ± 39.2	0	0	147.6 ± 37.5	0	0	0.57
Copper, mg/day	0.8	10	2.6 ± 0.9	1.3	0	2.7 ± 1.0	1.3	0	2.5 ± 0.9	2.5	0	0.23

[a] p-value for repeated measures ANOVA performed to assess variations in micronutrient intakes across trimesters. When no EAR or UL was established for a nutrient, the "–" is used instead of a 0. EAR: estimated average requirement; UL: upper intake limit; DFE: dietary folate equivalent; RAE: retinol activity equivalents; NE: niacin equivalent.

4. Discussion

Our prospective assessment of pregnant women's dietary intakes revealed a stability in energy and macronutrient intakes across trimesters. Most women exceeded their estimated requirements in terms of energy and protein in the first trimester but reported energy intakes below their needs later in pregnancy. We also found that diet alone may not be sufficient to provide adequate intakes for all micronutrients. Besides, when only food sources were considered, insufficient intakes of dietary fiber, vitamin D, folate, and iron were observed for a majority of women. Supplement use considerably improved the adequacy of micronutrient intakes among the pregnant women in our study sample, although excessive intakes were observed for iron, folic acid, and sodium.

Although it is recommended for pregnant women to increase their caloric intake as the pregnancy progresses [3], we found that there was a stability in energy intakes throughout pregnancy. Likewise, Abeysekera et al. [29] and Talai Rad et al. [30] as well as Moran et al. [18] found no significant changes in longitudinal caloric intakes of pregnant women. A prospective study by Vioque et al. conducted among Spanish pregnant women even observed a significant decrease in energy intakes (from the first to the third trimester) measured by a food frequency questionnaire (FFQ) [31]. Moreover, a recent meta-analysis of 18 studies by Jebeile et al. [32] reported little to no change in energy intake during pregnancy, which is in line with the stability we observed across trimesters. In light of their observations, Jebeile et al. [32] questioned the current caloric recommendations during pregnancy, suggesting they may be too high, but this affirmation should be further explored through studies that will focus on energy metabolism during pregnancy.

Although no variation in energy and macronutrient intakes was observed, most women exceeded their EER and EPR in the first trimester, in contrast with the third trimester, where a majority of women reported energy intakes below their EER. Kubota et al. [15] reported partially similar results, as they observed dietary intakes in the third trimester that were 900 kcal below the official Japanese recommendations. Since we do not have pre-pregnancy nutritional data, it is unknown whether the caloric excess observed is related to pregnancy itself or if it was already present before pregnancy. Augustine et al. [33] suggested that the process of «eating for two» associated with pregnancy occurs before the actual metabolic demand affects the mother. According to them, hormone-induced increase in dietary intakes early on in pregnancy could represent an adaptive response to the upcoming metabolic demand [33]. This could partially explain why our sample exceeded their EERs and EPRs as early as in the first trimester. The higher protein intakes observed in the first trimester also suggest that foods rich in protein (e.g., meat, dairy, legumes, etc.) may have contributed to the energy excess observed in early pregnancy, but this should be further investigated. Moreover, the questionnaire used to calculate PAL, the PPAQ, has been known to overestimate PAL in a small cohort of pregnant women [34]; therefore, the EERs calculated calculated within each trimester each trimester may have been overestimated. The use of a more precise method to measure our sample's PAL (e.g., an accelerometer), could have attenuated the gap between EIs and EERs in the third trimester but could have increased it in the first trimester.

In parallel with the energy and protein excess observed in the first trimester, we found that, in all trimesters, more than half of our study sample reported fat intakes as percentages of energy that exceeded the acceptable range of 20–35%. These results are similar to those of Dubois et al. [11] in which a third of the 1533 pregnant women studied had total fat intakes as a percentage of energy above the recommended range. Furthermore, a meta-analysis by Blumfield et al. [19] also found that studies set in Western regions reported mean fat intakes (as percentages of energy intakes) of 35.0% to 37.1% among pregnant women, in accordance with our results. Moreover, in our study, 20.3% to 24.1% of participants reported carbohydrate intakes as a percentage of energy below the recommendations, which is also similar to other North American studies [19]. However, the literature is still incomplete and unclear on the roles that each macronutrient plays in pregnant women's health [35]. Further research is therefore necessary to assess the impact of inadequate macronutrient intakes on maternal and fetal outcomes.

The suboptimal dietary intakes of fiber, vitamin D, folic acid, and iron observed in pregnant women from our study seem to be in line with the results of various authors [11,18,36–39]. Our results combined with those of other epidemiological studies thus suggest that food fortification policies and the use of a multivitamin during pregnancy are still necessary to reduce the risk of inadequate intake of micronutrients. In fact, our study showed that the use of dietary supplements greatly improved the adherence to micronutrient recommendations, as approximately 75% of all participants had total intakes above the EAR for all micronutrients. Dubois et al. [11] as well as Fayyaz et al. [40] reported similar results, especially regarding total iron and folate intakes. The insufficient intakes of dietary fiber observed in our study are in accordance with what Dubois et al. [11] reported, however, the relevance of these results and the impact of inadequate fiber intakes during pregnancy should be further investigated.

Most of our participants were supplement users and prenatal multivitamins were the most prevalent supplement taken by our study sample. It is important to mention that, although Health Canada recommends a prenatal multivitamin that contains 400 µg of folic acid and 16–20 mg of iron, close to all prenatal multivitamin supplements taken by our participants contained 1000 to 5000 µg of folic acid and 27 to 35 mg of iron (data not shown). Consequently, a majority of participants exceeded the UL for folic acid (1000 µg) in all trimesters and more than a third exceeded the UL for iron (45 mg) in the first and second trimesters. Dubois et al. [11] obtained similar results as they found that 90.4% and 32.4% of their participants had excessive folic acid and iron intakes, respectively, when dietary supplements were taken into account. Increased iron and folic acid intakes are indicated for women with conditions such as iron-deficiency anemia (iron) or for pregnant women at higher risk of giving birth to children with neural tube defects (folic acid) [41,42]. In our study, we do not have information regarding the number of women that were prescribed an iron supplement to prevent or to treat an iron-deficiency anemia. It is therefore impossible to know if the excessive iron intakes observed among our participants were due to anemia prevention or treatment. Moreover, it is important to mention that other nutrients, namely calcium, might decrease iron absorption, and thus observed total intakes of iron may not reflect the real iron status of our participants [43]. For these reasons, our results should be combined with direct assessment of iron status to evaluate the adequacy of our participant's iron intakes. Furthermore, results from a recent Canadian study suggest that although fortification policies improved the population's dietary intakes of folic acid, supplement users may be at risk of folic acid overconsumption [44]. To date, the implications of high folic acid intakes on pregnancy and prenatal health outcomes are not well understood and should therefore be further investigated [40,45,46].

Along with iron and folate, vitamin D was found to be one of the nutrients for which diet alone was insufficient to provide adequate intakes. The prevalence of inadequate intakes did decrease when dietary supplements were taken into account, but more than 20% of participants sill had total vitamin D intakes that were below the EAR, in all trimesters. Similar inadequacies were reported by Aghajafari et al. [37], as they found that 44% of their sample (*n* = 537 pregnant women) reported total vitamin D intakes (diet and supplements) that did not meet the Recommended Dietary Allowance (RDA) of 600 IU. Furthermore, despite the fact that more than half of their participants reported adequate daily vitamin D intakes (≥600 IU), Aghajafari et al. found that 20% of them were vitamin D-insufficient, according to the Endocrine Society and Osteoporosis Canada's definition of 75 nmol/L circulating 25-hydroxyvitamin D. [47,48]. Moreover, Hollis et al. [49] conducted a double-blind randomized clinical trial in 494 pregnant women and found that a vitamin D supplementation of 4000 IU/day was the most effective in achieving vitamin D sufficiency, in comparison with 400 and 2000 IU/day. In our study, prenatal multivitamins taken by pregnant women contained, depending on the brand of the multivitamin, between 250 and 600 IU of vitamin D (data not shown). This may not be adequate, according to Hollis et al. [49], to complement dietary intakes of all pregnant women. Nevertheless, evidence regarding vitamin D supplementation during pregnancy is not currently sufficient to support definite clinical recommendations, and the results of Hollis et al. should be interpreted with caution [50]. It would also be necessary to combine dietary assessment (food and supplements) with direct measurement of vitamin D status (i.e., circulating 25(OH)D) and sun exposure in order to accurately evaluate vitamin D adequacy during pregnancy [11,51].

To our knowledge, this is the first study to prospectively assess whether or not pregnant women met current Canadian nutritional recommendations. The use of a validated Web-based 24 h recall combined with a Web questionnaire on supplement use generated detailed information on dietary and total intakes during pregnancy. However, our study has some limitations, namely regarding the small size and the lack of representativeness of our study sample, since most pregnant women enrolled were Caucasians and of a higher socioeconomic status. The nutritional inadequacies observed among our study sample may therefore be greater among less educated and lower-income pregnant women. Nutritional adequacy of pregnant women of lower socioeconomic status should be further investigated. However, despite our small sample size, our results highlight the need for more prospective, population-based studies regarding pregnant women's dietary intakes, especially among lower income, less educated populations. Finally, our study did not measure circulating 25(OH)D in addition to iron and folate status, which limited our adequacy assessment of pregnant women's vitamin D, iron, and folate intakes.

5. Conclusions

In summary, we observed that, contrary to current recommendations, there was a stability in dietary intakes across trimesters, and thus most women exceeded their energy and protein requirements in the first trimester and had intakes below recommendations in the third trimester. The implications and possible causes of excessive energy and protein intakes in early pregnancy are not well documented and should be further investigated in association with gestational weight gain and other metabolic outcomes. The use of prenatal multivitamins and single nutrient supplements considerably improved iron, folate, and vitamin D adequacy, although excessive folic acid, iron, sodium, and niacin intakes were observed, and vitamin D inadequacies persisted for some pregnant women. Further research is needed to, firstly, evaluate the impact of high doses of folic acid on pregnancy and prenatal outcomes, and, secondly, to identify the dose of supplemental vitamin D necessary to achieve vitamin D sufficiency.

Author Contributions: All authors made substantial contributions to the conception and design of the manuscript, and all critically revised a first draft of the manuscript for important intellectual content. C.S. collected the data under the supervision of A.-S.M. and conducted primary statistical analyses of the data with the help of J.R., S.L., S.J.W., B.F.-B., C.G., and A.-S.M. All authors participated in the secondary analyses and interpretation of data. All authors gave their approval of the manuscript's final version to be published and therefore take public responsibility for the content of the manuscript. Finally, all authors agreed to be accountable for all aspects of the work.

Funding: The ANGE project is funded by the Danone Institute of Canada and by startup founds (Fonds de recherche du Québec-Santé et Fondation du CHU de Québec). All funding allowed the collection, analysis, and interpretation of data, but played no role in the writing of this manuscript.

Acknowledgments: We would like to acknowledge the valuable collaboration of trained dietician and graduate student Anne-Sophie Plante, as well as the research team that developed the R24W in collaboration with SL and JR: Benoît Lamarche, Louise Corneau, Catherine Laramée, and Simon Jacques.

Conflicts of Interest: The authors declare no conflict of interest.

References

1. Butte, N.F.; King, J.C. Energy requirements during pregnancy and lactation. *Public Health Nutr.* **2005**, *8*, 1010–1027. [CrossRef] [PubMed]
2. Fowles, E.R.; Fowles, S.L. Healthy eating during pregnancy: Determinants and supportive strategies. *J. Community Health Nurs.* **2008**, *25*, 138–152. [CrossRef] [PubMed]
3. Otten, J.J.; Hellwig, J.P.; Meyers, L.D. (Eds.) *Dietary Reference Intakes: The Essential Guide to Nutrient Requirements*; Institute of Medicine, National Academies Press: Washington, DC, USA, 2006.

4. Health Canada. *Prenatal Nutrition Guidelines for Health Professionals. Background on Canada's Food Guide*; Health Canada: Ottawa, ON, Canada, 2009.
5. Gernand, A.D.; Schulze, K.J.; Stewart, C.P.; West, K.P., Jr.; Christian, P. Micronutrient deficiencies in pregnancy worldwide: Health effects and prevention. *Nat. Rev. Endocrinol.* **2016**, *12*, 274–289. [CrossRef] [PubMed]
6. Morisset, A.S.; Weiler, H.A.; Dubois, L.; Ashley-Martin, J.; Shapiro, G.D.; Dodds, L.; Massarelli, I.; Vigneault, M.; Arbuckle, T.E.; Fraser, W.D. Rankings of iron, vitamin D, and calcium intakes in relation to maternal characteristics of pregnant Canadian women. *Appl. Physiol. Nutr. Metab.* **2016**, *41*, 749–757. [CrossRef] [PubMed]
7. Scholing, J.M.; Olthof, M.R.; Jonker, F.A.; Vrijkotte, T.G. Association between pre-pregnancy weight status and maternal micronutrient status in early pregnancy. *Public Health Nutr.* **2018**, 1–10. [CrossRef] [PubMed]
8. Breymann, C. Iron Deficiency Anemia in Pregnancy. *Semin. Hematol.* **2015**, *52*, 339–347. [CrossRef] [PubMed]
9. Goh, Y.I.; Koren, G. Folic acid in pregnancy and fetal outcomes. *J. Obstet. Gynaecol.* **2008**, *28*, 3–13. [CrossRef] [PubMed]
10. Martin, J.C.; Zhou, S.J.; Flynn, A.C.; Malek, L.; Greco, R.; Moran, L. The Assessment of Diet Quality and Its Effects on Health Outcomes Pre-pregnancy and during Pregnancy. *Semin. Reprod. Med.* **2016**, *34*, 83–92. [PubMed]
11. Dubois, L.; Diasparra, M.; Bédard, B.; Colapinto, C.K.; Fontaine-Bisson, B.; Morisset, A.S.; Tremblay, R.E.; Fraser, W.D. Adequacy of nutritional intake from food and supplements in a cohort of pregnant women in Quebec, Canada: The 3D Cohort Study (Design, Develop, Discover). *Am. J. Clin. Nutr.* **2017**, *106*, 541–548. [CrossRef] [PubMed]
12. Al Wattar, B.H.; Mylrea-Lowndes, B.; Morgan, C.; Moore, A.P.; Thangaratinam, S. Use of dietary assessment tools in randomized trials evaluating diet-based interventions in pregnancy: A systematic review of literature. *Curr. Opin. Obstet. Gynecol.* **2016**, *28*, 455–463. [CrossRef] [PubMed]
13. Kipnis, V.; Midthune, D.; Freedman, L.S.; Bingham, S.; Schatzkin, A.; Subar, A.; Carroll, R.J. Empirical evidence of correlated biases in dietary assessment instruments and its implications. *Am. J. Epidemiol.* **2001**, *153*, 394–403. [CrossRef] [PubMed]
14. Willet, W.C. *Nutritional Epidemiology*, 3rd ed.; Oxford University Press: New York, NY, USA, 2013.
15. Kubota, K.; Itoh, H.; Tasaka, M.; Naito, H.; Fukuoka, Y.; Muramatsu Kato, K.; Kohmura, Y.K.; Sugihara, K.; Kanayama, N. Changes of maternal dietary intake, bodyweight and fetal growth throughout pregnancy in pregnant Japanese women. *J. Obstet. Gynaecol. Res.* **2013**, *39*, 1383–1390. [CrossRef] [PubMed]
16. Lyu, L.C.; Hsu, Y.N.; Chen, H.F.; Lo, C.C.; Lin, C.L. Comparisons of four dietary assessment methods during pregnancy in Taiwanese women. *Taiwan. J. Obstet. Gynecol.* **2014**, *53*, 162–169. [CrossRef] [PubMed]
17. McGowan, C.A.; McAuliffe, F.M. Maternal dietary patterns and associated nutrient intakes during each trimester of pregnancy. *Public Health Nutr.* **2013**, *16*, 97–107. [CrossRef] [PubMed]
18. Moran, L.J.; Sui, Z.; Cramp, C.S.; Dodd, J.M. A decrease in diet quality occurs during pregnancy in overweight and obese women which is maintained post-partum. *Int. J. Obes. (Lond.)* **2013**, *37*, 704–711. [CrossRef] [PubMed]
19. Blumfield, M.L.; Hure, A.J.; Macdonald-Wicks, L.; Smith, R.; Collins, C.E. Systematic review and meta-analysis of energy and macronutrient intakes during pregnancy in developed countries. *Nutr. Rev.* **2012**, *70*, 322–336. [CrossRef] [PubMed]
20. Kopp-Hoolihan, L.E.; van Loan, M.D.; Wong, W.W.; King, J.C. Longitudinal assessment of energy balance in well-nourished, pregnant women. *Am. J. Clin. Nutr.* **1999**, *69*, 697–704. [CrossRef] [PubMed]
21. Jacques, S.; Lemieux, S.; Lamarche, B.; Laramée, C.; Corneau, L.; Lapointe, A.; Tessier-Grenier, M.; Robitaille, J. Development of a Web-Based 24-h Dietary Recall for a French-Canadian Population. *Nutrients* **2016**, *8*, 724. [CrossRef] [PubMed]
22. Moshfegh, A.J.; Rhodes, D.G.; Baer, D.J.; Murayi, T.; Clemens, J.C.; Rumpler, W.V.; Paul, D.R.; Sebastian, R.S.; Kuczynski, K.J.; Ingwersen, L.A.; et al. The US Department of Agriculture Automated Multiple-Pass Method reduces bias in the collection of energy intakes. *Am. J. Clin. Nutr.* **2008**, *88*, 324–332. [CrossRef] [PubMed]
23. Canadian Nutrient File (CNF). Available online: https://food-nutrition.canada.ca/cnf-fce/index-eng.jsp (accessed on 26 March 2018).
24. Savard, C.; Lemieux, S.; Lafrenière, J.; Laramée, C.; Robitaille, J.; Morisset, A.S. Validation of a self-administered web-based 24-hour dietary recall among pregnant women. *BMC Pregnancy Childbirth* **2018**, *18*, 112. [CrossRef] [PubMed]

25. Health Canada. Licensed Natural Health Product Database. Available online: https://health-products. canada.ca/lnhpd-bdpsnh/index-eng.jsp (accessed on 26 March 2018).

26. Chandonnet, N.; Saey, D.; Alméras, N.; Marc, I. French Pregnancy Physical Activity Questionnaire compared with an accelerometer cut point to classify physical activity among pregnant obese women. *PLoS ONE* **2012**, *7*, e38818. [CrossRef] [PubMed]

27. Chasan-taber, L.; Schmidt, M.D.; Roberts, D.E.; Hosmer, D.A.V.I.D.; Markenson, G.L.E.N.N.; Freedson, P.S. Development and validation of a Pregnancy Physical Activity Questionnaire. *Med. Sci. Sports Exerc.* **2004**, *36*, 1750–1760. [CrossRef] [PubMed]

28. Institute of Medicine (US) Subcommittee on Interpretation and Uses of Dietary Reference Intakes; Institute of Medicine (US) Standing Committee on the Scientific Evaluation of Dietary Reference Intakes. Application of DRIs for Group Diet Assessment. In *DRI Dietary Reference Intakes: Applications in Dietary Assessment*; National Academies Press: Washington, DC, USA, 2000.

29. Abeysekera, M.V.; Morris, J.A.; Davis, G.K.; O'sullivan, A.J. Alterations in energy homeostasis to favour adipose tissue gain: A longitudinal study in healthy pregnant women. *Aust. N. Z. J. Obstet. Gynaecol.* **2016**, *56*, 42–48. [CrossRef] [PubMed]

30. Rad, N.T.; Ritterath, C.; Siegmund, T.; Wascher, C.; Siebert, G.; Henrich, W.; Buhling, K.J. Longitudinal analysis of changes in energy intake and macronutrient composition during pregnancy and 6 weeks post-partum. *Arch. Gynecol. Obstet.* **2011**, *283*, 185–190.

31. Vioque, J.; Navarrete-Muñoz, E.M.; Gimenez-Monzó, D.; García-de-la-Hera, M.; Granado, F.; Young, I.S.; Ramón, R.; Ballester, F.; Murcia, M.; Rebagliato, M.; et al. Reproducibility and validity of a food frequency questionnaire among pregnant women in a Mediterranean area. *Nutr. J.* **2013**, *12*, 26. [CrossRef] [PubMed]

32. Jebeile, H.; Mijatovic, J.; Louie, J.C.Y.; Prvan, T.; Brand-Miller, J.C. A systematic review and metaanalysis of energy intake and weight gain in pregnancy. *Am. J. Obstet. Gynecol.* **2016**, *214*, 465–483. [CrossRef] [PubMed]

33. Augustine, R.A.; Ladyman, S.R.; Grattan, D.R. From feeding one to feeding many: Hormone-induced changes in bodyweight homeostasis during pregnancy. *J. Physiol.* **2008**, *586*, 387–397. [CrossRef] [PubMed]

34. Brett, K.E.; Wilson, S.; Ferraro, Z.M.; Adamo, K.B. Self-report Pregnancy Physical Activity Questionnaire overestimates physical activity. *Can. J. Public Health* **2015**, *106*, e297–e302. [CrossRef] [PubMed]

35. Tielemans, M.J.; Garcia, A.H.; Peralta Santos, A.; Bramer, W.M.; Luksa, N.; Luvizotto, M.J.; Moreira, E.; Topi, G.; De Jonge, E.A.; Visser, T.L.; Voortman, T. Macronutrient composition and gestational weight gain: A systematic review. *Am. J. Clin. Nutr.* **2016**, *103*, 83–99. [CrossRef] [PubMed]

36. Roy, A.; Evers, S.E.; Campbell, M.K. Dietary supplement use and iron, zinc and folate intake in pregnant women in London, Ontario. *Chronic Dis. Inj. Can.* **2012**, *32*, 76–83. [PubMed]

37. Aghajafari, F.; Field, C.J.; Kaplan, B.J.; Rabi, D.M.; Maggiore, J.A.; O'Beirne, M.; Hanley, D.A.; Eliasziw, M.; Dewey, D.; Weinberg, A.; et al. The Current Recommended Vitamin D Intake Guideline for Diet and Supplements During Pregnancy Is Not Adequate to Achieve Vitamin D Sufficiency for Most Pregnant Women. *PLoS ONE* **2016**, *11*, e0157262. [CrossRef] [PubMed]

38. Kocyłowski, R.; Lewicka, I.; Grzesiak, M.; Gaj, Z.; Sobańska, A.; Poznaniak, J.; von Kaisenberg, C.; Suliburska, J. Assessment of dietary intake and mineral status in pregnant women. *Arch. Gynecol. Obstet.* **2018**, *297*, 1433–1440. [CrossRef] [PubMed]

39. Blumfield, M.L.; Hure, A.J.; Macdonald-Wicks, L.; Smith, R.; Collins, C.E. A systematic review and meta-analysis of micronutrient intakes during pregnancy in developed countries. *Nutr. Rev.* **2013**, *71*, 118–132. [CrossRef] [PubMed]

40. Fayyaz, F.; Wang, F.; Jacobs, R.L.; O'Connor, D.L.; Bell, R.C.; Field, C.J.; APrON Study Team. Folate, vitamin B12, and vitamin B6 status of a group of high socioeconomic status women in the Alberta Pregnancy Outcomes and Nutrition (APrON) cohort. *Appl. Physiol. Nutr. Metab.* **2014**, *39*, 1402–1408. [CrossRef] [PubMed]

41. Wilson, R.D.; Audibert, F.; Brock, J.A.; Carroll, J.; Cartier, L.; Gagnon, A.; Johnson, J.A.; Langlois, S.; Murphy-Kaulbeck, L.; Okun, N.; Pastuck, M. Pre-conception Folic Acid and Multivitamin Supplementation for the Primary and Secondary Prevention of Neural Tube Defects and Other Folic Acid-Sensitive Congenital Anomalies. *J. Obstet. Gynaecol. Can.* **2015**, *37*, 534–552. [CrossRef]

42. Peña-Rosas, J.P.; De-Regil, L.M.; Dowswell, T.; Viteri, F.E. Daily oral iron supplementation during pregnancy. *Cochrane Database Syst. Rev.* **2015**, CD004736. [CrossRef] [PubMed]

43. Hallberg, L.; Rossander-Hulten, L.; Brune, M.; Gleerup, A. Calcium and iron absorption: Mechanism of action and nutritional importance. *Eur. J. Clin. Nutr.* **1992**, *46*, 317–327. [PubMed]

44. Mudryj, A.N.; de Groh, M.; Aukema, H.M.; Yu, N. Folate intakes from diet and supplements may place certain Canadians at risk for folic acid toxicity. *Br. J. Nutr.* **2016**, *116*, 1236–1245. [CrossRef] [PubMed]

45. Barua, S.; Kuizon, S.; Junaid, M.A. Folic acid supplementation in pregnancy and implications in health and disease. *J. Biomed. Sci.* **2014**, *21*, 77. [CrossRef] [PubMed]

46. De Boer, A.; Bast, A.; Godschalk, R. Dietary supplement intake during pregnancy; better safe than sorry? *Regul. Toxicol. Pharmacol.* **2018**, *95*, 442–447. [CrossRef] [PubMed]

47. Hanley, D.A.; Cranney, A.; Jones, G.; Whiting, S.J.; Leslie, W.D.; Cole, D.E.; Atkinson, S.A.; Josse, R.G.; Feldman, S.; Kline, G.A.; Rosen, C. Vitamin D in adult health and disease: A review and guideline statement from Osteoporosis Canada. *CMAJ* **2010**, *182*, E610–E618. [CrossRef] [PubMed]

48. Holick, M.F.; Binkley, N.C.; Bischoff-Ferrari, H.A.; Gordon, C.M.; Hanley, D.A.; Heaney, R.P.; Murad, M.H.; Weaver, C.M. Evaluation, treatment, and prevention of vitamin D deficiency: An Endocrine Society clinical practice guideline. *J. Clin. Endocrinol. Metab.* **2011**, *96*, 1911–1930. [CrossRef] [PubMed]

49. Hollis, B.W.; Johnson, D.; Hulsey, T.C.; Ebeling, M.; Wagner, C.L. Vitamin D supplementation during pregnancy: Double-blind, randomized clinical trial of safety and effectiveness. *J. Bone Miner. Res.* **2011**, *26*, 2341–2357. [CrossRef] [PubMed]

50. Harvey, N.C.; Holroyd, C.; Ntani, G.; Javaid, K.; Cooper, P.; Moon, R.; Cole, Z.; Tinati, T.; Godfrey, K.; Dennison, E.; Bishop, N.J. Vitamin D supplementation in pregnancy: A systematic review. *Health Technol. Assess.* **2014**, *18*, 1–190. [CrossRef] [PubMed]

51. Savard, C.; Gagnon, C.; Morisset, A.S. Disparities in the timing and measurement methods to assess vitamin D status during pregnancy: A Narrative Review. *Int. J. Vitam. Nutr. Res.* **2018**, in press.

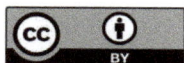

nutrients

MDPI

Article

Single Nucleotide Polymorphisms in Vitamin D Receptor Gene Affect Birth Weight and the Risk of Preterm Birth: Results From the "Mamma & Bambino" Cohort and A Meta-Analysis

Martina Barchitta [1], Andrea Maugeri [1], Maria Clara La Rosa [1], Roberta Magnano San Lio [1], Giuliana Favara [1], Marco Panella [2], Antonio Cianci [2] and Antonella Agodi [1,*]

[1] Department of Medical and Surgical Sciences and Advanced Technologies "GF Ingrassia", University of Catania, via S. Sofia, 87, 95123 Catania, Italy; martina.barchitta@unict.it (M.B.); andreamaugeri88@gmail.com (A.M.); mariclalarosa@gmail.com (M.C.L.R.); robimagnano@gmail.com (R.M.S.L.); giuliana.favara@gmail.com (G.F.)

[2] Department of General Surgery and Medical Surgical Specialties, University of Catania, Via S. Sofia, 78, 95123 Catania, Italy; mpanella@unict.it (M.P.); acianci@unict.it (A.C.)

* Correspondence: agodia@unict.it

Received: 24 July 2018; Accepted: 25 August 2018; Published: 27 August 2018

check for updates

Abstract: The effect of vitamin D receptor gene (VDR) polymorphisms on adverse pregnancy outcomes—including preterm birth (PTB), low birth weight and small for gestational age—is currently under debate. We investigated 187 mother-child pairs from the Italian "Mamma & Bambino" cohort to evaluate the association of maternal VDR polymorphisms—BsmI, ApaI, FokI and TaqI—with neonatal anthropometric measures and the risk of PTB. To corroborate our results, we conducted a meta-analysis of observational studies. For the FokI polymorphism, we showed that gestational duration and birth weight decreased with increasing number of A allele ($p = 0.040$ and $p = 0.010$, respectively). Compared to the GG and GA genotypes, mothers who carried the AA genotype exhibited higher PTB risk (OR = 12.049; 95% CI = 2.606–55.709; $p = 0.001$) after adjusting for covariates. The meta-analysis confirmed this association under the recessive model (OR = 3.67, 95%CI 1.18–11.43), and also pointed out the protective effect of BsmI polymorphism against the risk of PTB under the allelic (A vs. G: OR = 0.74; 95%CI 0.59–0.93) and recessive (AA vs. GG + AG: OR = 0.62; 95%CI 0.43–0.89) models. Our results suggest the association between some maternal VDR polymorphisms with neonatal anthropometric measures and the risk of PTB.

Keywords: pregnancy; vitamin D; gestational duration; birth cohort

1. Introduction

Adverse pregnancy outcomes continue to be major Public Health problems in spite of improvements in health care [1–3]. Among these, preterm birth (PTB) represents the first cause of death among newborns and the second among children under five years [4]. Since the World Health Organization (WHO) estimated that 15 million of children prematurely born each year—it means more than one out of ten infants—novel strategies and guidelines should be designed and validated to help prevent PTB. The major risk factors of PTB are certainly maternal age, short inter-pregnancy interval, multiple gestation, drug abuse, smoking, vaginal dysbiosis and infections, low maternal pre-pregnancy weight or inadequate gestational weight gain [5–8]. However, the effect of genetic susceptibility has been also well recognized [9], with novel fetal and maternal genomic variants which in turn affect both intrauterine environment, pregnancy duration and fetal growth [10]. It has been estimated that approximately 32 million low birth weight (LBW) or small for gestational age (SGA) infants are born annually, with 96.5% of them in developing countries [11]. Approximately two-thirds of the risk of adverse pregnancy outcomes depend on maternal habits, with maternal nutrition playing a key role during the preconception and gestational periods [12]. However, uncovering the main genetic risk factors of adverse pregnancy outcomes remains one of the main challenges for Public Health, since they conferred about a third of this risk [13–15].

Overall, vitamin D is crucial for the maintenance of adult health [16] and its deficiency—especially during pregnancy—is associated with potential adverse outcomes for both mothers and children [17]. In humans, most of Vitamin D is provided by the endogenous cutaneous synthesis of pre-vitamin D3, which is derived from 7-dehydrocholesterol through the exposure to ultraviolet radiation [18]. The best sources of vitamin D are the flesh of fatty fish (i.e., salmon, tuna, and mackerel) and fish liver oils, while small amounts of vitamin D are found in beef liver, cheese, and egg yolks [19,20]. Vitamin D in these foods is primarily in the form of vitamin D3 [21]. In U.S.A. and Canada, fortified foods provide most of the vitamin D in the D3 form [19,22]. While Vitamin D3 represents almost 95% vitamin D serum levels [23], a less active form, known as Vitamin D2, is also provided by dietary sources and supplements [24]. Therefore, serum levels of 25-hydroxylated vitamin D2+D3 (25OHD) represent the vitamin D pool of the body. During pregnancy, the fetus is entirely dependent on maternal sources of vitamin D, which also regulates placental function [18]. Several observational studies showed that maternal vitamin D deficiency may influence mother and neonatal outcomes, including recurrent pregnancy losses, preeclampsia, gestational diabetes, PTB, LBW and SGA [25]. However, as concluded by recent systematic reviews and meta-analyses, it is currently not clear if adequate dietary intake and/or supplementation of vitamin D may reduce the risk of adverse pregnancy outcomes [25–28]. Inconclusive results could be partially explained by heterogeneity in study design, exposure variables, outcomes of interest, study setting and participants.

In this scenario, increasing interest concerns the effect of genetic variants affecting vitamin D metabolism and functions. Vitamin D activity is mediated by the vitamin D receptor (VDR), a nuclear receptor which acts as a high-affinity ligand-activated transcription factor [29]. VDR gene—located on the chromosome 12q12–14—is highly expressed in several human tissues including skin epithelium, osteoblasts and chondrocytes, muscles, cells from the immune system and placenta [30]. The ligand-bound VDR forms a heterodimer with nuclear retinoid X receptor (RXR) [31], which recognizes vitamin D response elements (VDRE) in the promoter regions of vitamin D target genes and recruits co-factors to modulate gene transcription [32]. Recently, some studies proposed the potential association between VDR polymorphisms and the risk of adverse pregnancy outcomes, such as PTB, LBW and SGA births [9,33–42]. In this area of research, BsmI (rs1544410), ApaI (rs7975232), FokI (rs2228570) and TaqI (rs731236) polymorphisms are the most commonly investigated: while TaqI and FokI consist of a single base change (A to G and G to A in exons 9 and 2, respectively), BsmI and ApaI are located in the last intron of the sequence and result from a single base change (G to A and A to C, respectively). However, evidence of an association between VDR polymorphisms and adverse pregnancy outcomes is currently weak and not convincing, with high heterogeneity across studies [43]. To explore the effect of preconception, perinatal and early life exposure on maternal and infant health—with particular focus on the interaction between epigenetic biomarkers of health and aging, diet and lifestyles [44–48]—we recently designed the prospective "Mamma & Bambino" study, which enrols mother-child pairs during pregnancy.

In the present study we used data and samples from this cohort to evaluate the association of maternal VDR polymorphisms (i.e., BsmI, ApaI, FokI and TaqI) with neonatal anthropometric measures and the risk of PTB, even considering dietary intake of vitamin D. Then, we carried out a systematic review evaluating the effect of VDR polymorphisms on PTB risk and on neonatal anthropometric measures. Finally, we corroborated our results by pooling them with those reported by previous studies through a meta-analysis.

2. Materials and Methods

2.1. Study Design

The "Mamma & Bambino" cohort is an ongoing Italian birth cohort designed to explore the effect of preconception, perinatal and early life exposure on maternal and infant health (further information can be found at http://www.birthcohorts.net). During the prenatal genetic counselling, at gestational week 4–20 (mean = 16 weeks), pregnant women referred to the Azienda Ospedaliera Universitaria "Policlinico-Vittorio Emanuele", Catania (Italy) were invited to participate. This study was carried out in accordance with the Declaration of Helsinki and the protocol was approved by the ethics committee of the involved institution. All subjects were fully informed of the purpose and procedures and gave written informed consent. In this cohort, information on sociodemographic and lifestyle data are collected by trained epidemiologists using a structured questionnaire. Educational level is classified as low (primary school, i.e., ≤8 years of school) and high (high school education or greater, i.e., >8 years of school). Women are also classified as employed or unemployed (including students and housewives). Smoking status is classified as no smoking (including ex-smokers) and current smoking. Pre-pregnancy body mass index (BMI) is calculated as weight (kg) divided by height (m^2), based on criteria from the WHO [49]. According to the Institute of Medicine (IOM) recommendations, we define adequate gestational weight gain (GWG) as follows: 12.5–18 kg (underweight), 11.5–16 kg (normal weight), 7–11.5 kg (overweight), and at least 5–9 kg (obese) [50]. Type of delivery, intrauterine foetal death, congenital malformations and plurality are also recorded at delivery. Biological samples are collected from both the mothers (peripheral blood) and the children (amniotic fluid and cord blood). Furthermore, a two-year follow-up is conducted to collect information on mother-child lifestyle and health status.

In the current analysis we included mother-child pairs with complete data on sociodemographic characteristics, lifestyle and vitamin D intake, pregnancy outcomes and maternal VDR genotype distributions. Primary outcomes were gestational duration and PTB, defined as spontaneous delivery before 37 weeks. Secondary outcomes were birth weight and length; birthweight was classified as LBW (birthweight < 2.5 kg) and macrosomia (birthweight ≥ 4.0 kg); birthweight for gestational age was defined as SGA, AGA or LGA according to sex-specific national reference charts [51]. Mother-child pairs with pre-existing medical conditions (i.e., autoimmune and/or chronic diseases), pregnancy complications (i.e., preeclampsia, hypertension and diabetes), pre-term induced delivery or caesarean section, intrauterine foetal death, plurality and congenital malformations were all excluded.

2.1.1. VDR Genotyping

Maternal DNA was extracted from peripheral blood samples using QIAamp DNA Mini Kit according to the manufacturer protocol (Qiagen, Milan, Italy). VDR polymorphisms were genotyped using the following commercially available TaqMan SNP Genotyping Assays (Applied Biosystem, Foster City, CA, USA): ApaI rs7975232 (C_28977635_10), TaqI rs731236 (C_2404008_10), BsmI rs1544410 (C_8716062_10), FokI rs2228570 (C_12060045_20). All reactions were performed in triplicate on the QuantStudio™ 7 Flex Real-Time PCR System (Applied Biosystem, Foster City, CA, USA) deploying conditions set by the manufacturer. Allele determination was carried out using QuantStudio™ 7 Flex System Software (Applied Biosystem, Foster City, CA, USA).

2.1.2. Assessment of Vitamin D Intake

Vitamin D intake was assessed by a validated 95-item semi-quantitative Food Frequency Questionnaire (FFQ) as described elsewhere [52]. In brief, women were asked to report the frequency of consumption (twelve categories from "almost never" to "two or more times a day") and portion size (small, medium or large) of each food item, using and indicative photograph atlas. Food intakes were calculated by multiplying the frequency of consumption with the daily portion size of each food item. Vitamin D intake was calculated using the USDA Nutrient Database (http://ndb.nal.usda.gov/)

adapted to the Italian food consumption. The use of multimineral/multivitamin supplements containing vitamin D was recorded, but the vitamin D intake was based only on food sources, as the FFQ was not designed to ascertain the quantification of vitamin D intake by supplementation.

2.1.3. Statistical Analyses

Statistical analyses were conducted using SPSS software (IBM Corp. Released 2013. IBM SPSS Statistics for Windows, Version 22.0. Armonk, NY, USA). Descriptive statistics were used to characterize the study population, using frequency, mean and standard deviation (SD), or median and interquartile range (IQR). The Chi-square test was performed to determine if geno-type distributions in mothers with full-term delivery were deviated from the Hardy-Weinberg Equilibrium (HWE). Prior to analysis, the normal distribution of all variables was checked using the Kolmogorov-Smirnov test. Based on skewed distribution, comparisons of maternal and infant quantitative variables across VDR genotypes were analysed using the Mann-Whitney U test or the Kruskal-Wallis test. Categorical variables were compared using the Chi-squared test. Linear and binary regression models were applied to evaluate the associations of VDR polymorphisms with primary and secondary outcomes, using the non-mutated genotypes as reference. Regression models were adjusted for age, smoking, educational level, employment status, pre-gestational BMI, GWG, vitamin D intake, use of vitamin D supplements, type of delivery and parity. Post-hoc statistical power analysis was performed using Epi Info™ software (version 7; CDC, Atlanta, GA, USA). All statistical tests were two-sided, and p values < 0.05 were considered statistically significant.

2.2. Systematic Review and Meta-Analysis

2.2.1. Search Strategy

Two of the Authors carried out a systematic literature search in the PubMed-Medline and Web of Science databases to identify relevant epidemiological studies, investigating the association of BsmI, ApaI, FokI and TaqI polymorphism with neonatal anthropometric measures and incidence of PTB, LBW and SGA births. The search strategy comprised the terms (Vitamin D receptor OR VDR) AND (variation OR polymorphism OR mutations OR SNP) AND (Preterm Birth OR birthweight OR birth weight OR birth length OR Low Birth Weight OR Intrauterine Growth Retardation OR Fetal Growth Retardation OR Small for Gestational Age). The databases were searched from inception to February 2018 without language restriction; abstracts and unpublished studies were not included. Moreover, the reference lists from selected articles, including relevant review papers, were searched to identify all appropriate studies. The preferred reporting items for systematic reviews and meta-analysis (PRISMA) guidelines were followed.

2.2.2. Selection Criteria

Two of the Authors independently assessed the retrieved articles and any inconsistencies were resolved through discussion. Studies included were consistent with the following criteria: (i) observational studies or randomized control trials (RCTs) (ii) on pregnant women of any gestational age (iii) without pregnancy complications, (iv) focusing on the association of FokI, ApaI, TaqI and BsmI VDR polymorphisms with PTB, LBW, and SGA. Moreover, (v) studies were selected if they provide sufficient information on the numbers or genotype frequencies in cases and controls in order to estimate odds ratios (ORs) and 95% confidence intervals (95% Cis). By contrast, the exclusion criteria were as follow: (i) systematic reviews or meta-analyses; (ii) abstracts and unpublished studies; (iii) studies with insufficient or lack of data to estimate ORs and 95% CIs, after attempting to contact the corresponding authors via e-mail; (iv) investigating the association with other VDR polymorphisms (v) or with other adverse pregnancy outcomes; (vi) studies with no control group.

2.2.3. Study Selection and Data Extraction

Two of the Authors independently extracted the following information: first Author's last name, year of publication, country where the study was performed, ethnicity and number of participants, sample type, phenotype of the cases evaluated, genotyping method, genotype distributions in cases and controls, and p-values for HWE in controls. If additional data were needed, the Authors of retrieved articles were contacted. Primary outcome was PTB since lack of data and inconsistency of reported outcomes avoided the quantitative analysis for birthweight, birth length, LBW and SGA.

2.2.4. Procedures of Meta-Analysis

Strength of association between VDR polymorphisms and PTB was estimated as ORs (95% CIs) under the allelic model (2 vs. 1), the dominant model (22 and 12 vs. 11) and the recessive model (22 vs. 11 and 12). The significance of pooled OR was determined by the Z test. Heterogeneity across studies was measured using the Q test, considering significant statistical heterogeneity as $p < 0.1$. As the Q test only indicates the presence of heterogeneity and not its magnitude, we also reported the I^2 statistic, which estimates the percentage of outcome variability that can be attributed to heterogeneity across studies. An I^2 value of 0% denotes no observed heterogeneity, whereas, 25% is "low", 50% is "moderate" and 75% is "high" heterogeneity [53]. We also estimated the between-study variance using tau-squared (t) statistics [54]. According to heterogeneity across studies, we used the fixed-effects model (Mantel-Haenszel method) when heterogeneity was negligible or the random-effects models (DerSimonian-Laird method) when heterogeneity was significant. The presence of publication bias was investigated by Begg's test and Egger's regression asymmetry test [55,56]. Except for the Q test, $p < 0.05$ was considered statistically significant, and all tests were 2-sided. All statistical analyses were performed using the Review Manager software (Version 5.3. Copenhagen: The Nordic Cochrane Centre, the Cochrane Collaboration, 2014).

3. Results

3.1. "Mamma & Bambino" Cohort

From the "Mamma & Bambino" cohort, 187 women aged 15–50 years (median = 37 years) were enrolled at a median gestational age of 16 weeks (IQR = 4). According to pre-gestational BMI and GWG we identified 30.9% and 27.1% who exhibited reduced or excessive GWG, respectively. In general, gestational duration was 39 weeks (IQR = 2) and 55.1% of deliveries were natural. Median birth length and weight were 50.0 cm (IQR = 2) and 3.2 Kg (IQR = 0.6), respectively. Approximately 8% of new-borns were underweight while 7.5% was diagnosed with macrosomia. According to sex-specific national reference charts [51], most of new-borns were AGA (80.2%), while the proportion of SGA and LGA were 8% and 11.8%, respectively. Only 10.7% of women reported the use of multimineral/multivitamin supplements containing vitamin D. Notably, vitamin D intake was not associated with neonatal anthropometric measures nor with PTB risk (Table 1). Table 1 also shows the comparison between mothers with PTB (n = 17; 9%) and full-term delivery (n = 170, 91%). No differences were evident for maternal socio-demographic characteristics, pre-gestational BMI, GWG, use of vitamin D supplements and lifestyle. As expected, PTB new-borns exhibited lower birth length (47.5 cm vs. 50.0 cm; $p < 0.001$) and weight (2.44 kg vs. 3.2 kg; $p < 0.001$), with a higher proportion of underweight compared to full-term new-borns (58.8% vs. 2.9%; $p < 0.001$).

Table 1. Population characteristics and comparison between preterm and full-term births.

Characteristics	Study Population (*n* = 187)	PTB (*n* = 17)	Full-Term (*n* = 170)	*p*-Value
Age, years [a]	37.0 (4)	37.0 (5)	38.0 (4)	0.648
Gestational age at enrolment, weeks	16.0 (4)	16.0 (4)	16.0 (4)	0.691
Educational level (% low-medium)	13.9%	5.9%	14.7%	0.316
Employment status (% employed)	55.6%	47.1%	56.5%	0.456
Smoking (% current smokers)	18.3%	5.8%	19.5%	0.165
Pre-gestational nutritional status				
Underweight	8.1%	11.8%	7.7%	0.522
Normal weight	65.6%	58.8%	66.3%	
Overweight	17.2%	11.8%	17.8%	
Obese	9.1%	17.6%	8.3%	
GWG, kg [a]	12.0 (7)	11.0 (10)	12.0 (6.9)	0.630
GWG classification				
Reduced	30.9%	35.3%	30.5%	0.903
Adequate	42%	41.2%	42.1%	
Excessive	27.1%	23.5%	27.4%	
Vitamin D intake, µg/day [a]	3.7 (3.5)	3.7 (4.3)	3.1 (3.6)	0.808
Vitamin D supplements (% users)	10.7%	5.9%	11.2%	0.501
Gestational duration, weeks	39.0 (2)	35.5 (2)	39.0 (2)	<0.001
Sex (% male)	50.3%	47.1%	50.6%	0.781
Birth weight, kg [a]	3.2 (0.6)	2.44 0.5)	3.2 (0.6)	<0.001
Birth length, cm [a]	50.0 (2)	47.5 (4)	50.0 (2)	<0.001
Type of delivery				
Natural	55.1%	47.1%	55.9%	0.486
Caesarean section	44.9%	52.9%	44.1%	
Underweight (%)	8%	58.8%	2.9%	<0.001
Macrosomia (%)	7.5%	0%	8.2%	0.219
Weight for gestational age				
SGA	8%	5.9%	8.2%	0.283
AGA	80.2%	70.6%	81.2%	
LGA	11.8%	23.5%	10.6%	

[a] Data reported as median (IQR). Abbreviations: IQR, interquartile range; PTB, preterm birth; GWG, gestational weight gain; SGA, small for gestational age; AGA, adequate for gestational age; LGA, large for gestational age.

Figure 1A shows the distributions of VDR genotypes in the study population; notably, only FokI and TaqI VDR polymorphisms were in HWE. The comparison of neonatal anthropometric measures across TaqI genotypes showed that birth weight increased with increasing number of G allele (AA = 3.2 kg vs. AG = 3.2 kg vs. GG = 3.4; *p* = 0.020). However, we failed in confirming this difference after adjusting for covariates. The comparison of maternal and neonatal characteristics across FokI genotypes showed that gestational duration and birth weight decreased with increasing number of A allele (*p* = 0.040 and *p* = 0.010, respectively). Accordingly, the proportion of PTB increased with increasing number of A allele (GG = 5.2% vs. AG = 8.3% vs. AA = 33.3%; *p* = 0.001), whereas no statistically significant differences were reported for BsmI, ApaI and TaqI (Figure 1B). In line with this evidence, we demonstrated that the risk of PTB increased with the number of A allele both in the age-adjusted (OR = 3.010; 95% CI = 1.457–6.215; *p* = 003) and in the multivariable-adjusted models (OR = 4.015; 95% CI = 1.649–9.771; *p* = 0.002). Particularly, compared to the GG and GA genotypes, mothers who carried the AA genotype exhibited a higher PTB risk both in the age-adjusted (OR = 7.389; 95% CI = 2.308-23.660; *p* = 0.001) and in the multivariable-adjusted models (OR = 12.049; 95% CI = 2.606–55.709; *p* = 0.001).

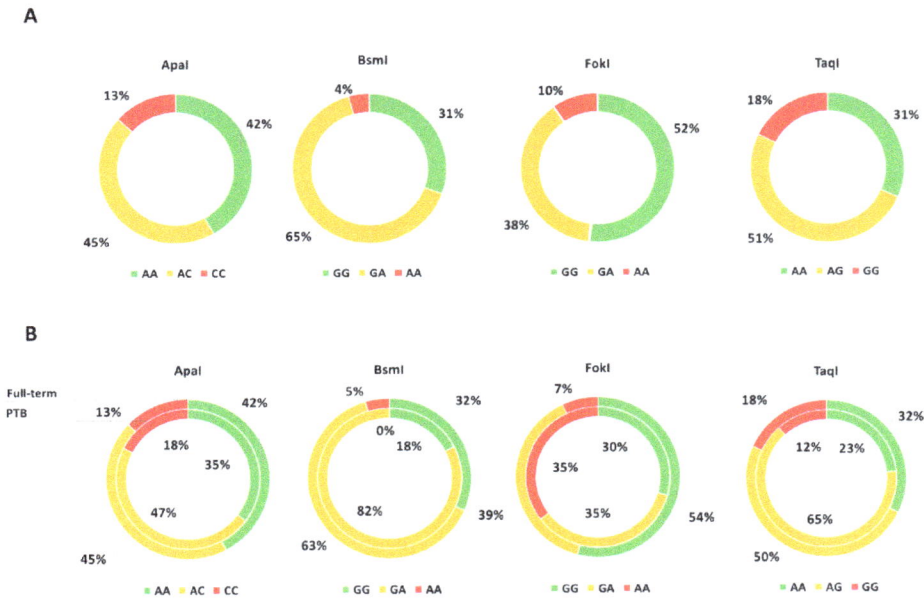

Figure 1. (**A**) Genotype Distribution of vitamin D receptor gene (VDR) Polymorphisms and (**B**) comparison between preterm births (PTB, inner ring) and full-term births (outer ring).

3.2. Systematic Review

3.2.1. Study Characteristics

The detailed steps of study selection are given as a PRISMA flow diagram in Figure 2. A total of 67 articles were retrieved from the databases and 18 duplicates were excluded. After reading titles and/or abstracts, 25 articles were excluded while 24 underwent full-text screening. Based on selection criteria we excluded 13 studies, whereas 11 studies were included in the systematic review. No RCTs focusing on the association of VDR polymorphisms with PTB, LBW, and SGA were found and thus, only observational studies were included.

A total of 5 studies were from European countries [9,36,38,40,42], 4 from America [33,35,37,41], and 1 from Asia [34] and Australia [39], respectively. Overall, sample sizes ranged from 189 to 615 mothers and from 90 to 506 infants, respectively. The most reported outcome was PTB (*n* = 4) [9,33,34,36], while 3 studies investigated neonatal anthropometric measures using birth weight [37], LBW [35] or SGA [41] as primary outcome. Two studies collected both maternal and cord blood samples [34,36], while 5 and 3 studies genotyped VDR polymorphisms in cord blood [38–42] or maternal blood samples [9,33,37], respectively; only Workalemahu et al. collected placental samples [35]. Given that the majority analysed more than one polymorphism, FokI was analysed by 7 studies [33–37,39,41], BsmI by 8 studies [9,34,36,38–42], ApaI by 5 studies [9,34,36,37,39,40] and TaqI by 7 studies [9,34,36–40]. The most common genotyping method was restriction fragment length polymorphism analysis (RFLP) (*n* = 6) [34,36–40,42], followed by TaqMan SNP Genotyping Assays (*n* = 4) [9,33,37,41] and Sequenom MassARRAY (*n* = 1) [35].

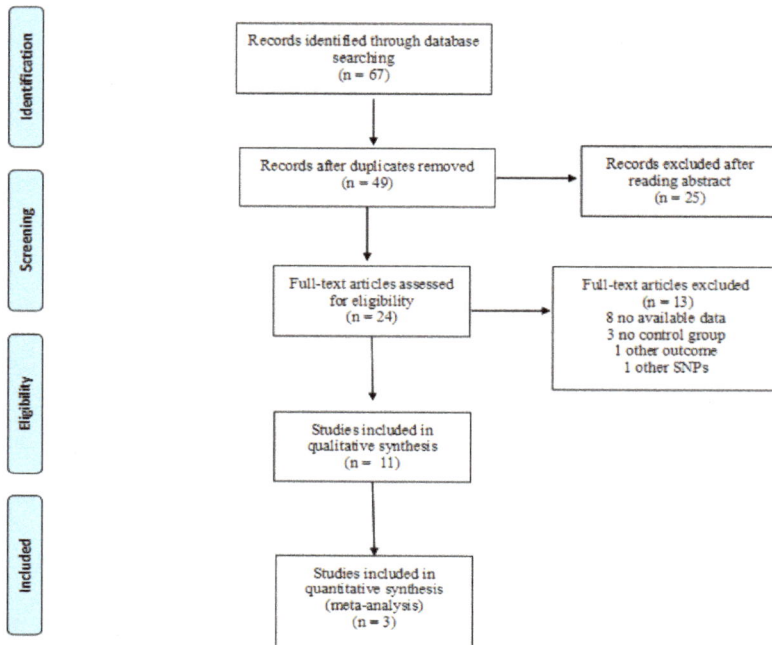

Figure 2. Flow diagram of study selection.

3.2.2. VDR Polymorphisms and Neonatal Anthropometric Measures

In 2011, Swamy and colleagues conducted a prospective study on 615 pregnant women, evaluating the effect of 38 VDR polymorphisms on several birth outcomes. In brief, they showed that 8 of 38 SNPs examined—including ApaI—were significantly associated with birth weight in black but not in white women [37]. In the same year, Silvano and colleagues studied 97 pre-pubertal singleton children from 0 to 12 years to assess clinical and biochemical phenotypes that better characterize SGA children who failed to achieve postnatal catch-up growth. At the baseline, they did not observe difference in BsmI and FokI genotype distributions across categories of birth weight for gestational age [41]. Consistently with our results, the study by Workalemahu et al.—investigating the effect of placental VDR polymorphisms on birth size in 506 mother-child pairs—demonstrated that birth weight decreased with increasing number of A allele of the FokI polymorphism [35].

3.2.3. VDR Polymorphisms and PTB Risk

Manzon and colleagues genotyped VDR polymorphisms in both maternal and cord blood samples of 33 PTB and 98 full-term delivery [36]. In line with our results, they concluded that women who carried the A allele of FokI were at higher risk of PTB than those who carried the G allele. By contrast, women who carried the T allele of TaqI polymorphism exhibited a lower risk of PTB [36] compared to those with non-mutated allele [36]. However, using a logistic regression model they observed that only maternal FokI variant was associated with the risk of PTB. More recently, the study by Javorsky and colleagues—comparing104 women with PTB to 85 with full-term delivery—confirmed that maternal FokI polymorphism was associated with a higher risk of PTB [33]. Next, Rosenfeld and colleagues added to this knowledge, demonstrating that the proportion of women with PTB decreased with increasing number of A allele of maternal BsmI polymorphism, after adjusting for some confounders [34]. Interestingly, among women with previous history of spontaneous miscarriage, the risk of PTB was higher if their newborns carried the non-mutated allele of BsmI or the mutated allele of ApaI [34].

3.2.4. Meta-Analyses of the Association between VDR Polymorphisms and PTB Risk

As demonstrated by post-hoc statistical power analysis, only the study of the association between FokI polymorphism and PTB reached a statistical power of at least 80%, with a significance level of 0.05. Thus, to summarize evidence about the association between maternal VDR polymorphisms and PTB, we pooled our results with those reported by three previously published articles [9,33,34] (Table 2). For the ApaI polymorphism, we pooled our results with those reported by Baczyńska-Strzecha et al. and Rosenfeld et al. [9,34]. The Q-test and I^2 statistics showed no significant heterogeneity across studies under the allelic ($p = 0.41$; $I^2 = 0\%$), dominant ($p = 0.19$; $I^2 = 40\%$) and recessive ($p = 0.61$; $I^2 = 0\%$) models. Using the fixed effect model, the meta-analysis showed no association of ApaI with PTB under the allelic model (C vs. A: OR = 0.89, 95%CI 0.71–1.12), dominant (CC + AC vs. AA: OR = 0.73, 95%CI 0.53–1.2) and recessive model (CC vs. AA + AC: OR = 1.20, 95%CI 0.81–1.77) (Figure 3).

For the BsmI polymorphism, we pooled our results with those reported by Baczyńska-Strzecha et al. and Rosenfeld et al. [9,34]. The Q-test and I^2 statistics showed no significant heterogeneity across studies under the allelic ($p = 0.31$; $I^2 = 15\%$), dominant ($p = 0.18$; $I^2 = 42\%$) and recessive ($p = 0.97$; $I^2 = 0\%$) models. Using the fixed effect model, the meta-analysis showed a significant negative association with PTB under the allelic (A vs. G: OR = 0.74, 95%CI 0.59–0.93) and recessive (AA vs. GG + AG: OR = 0.62, 95%CI 0.43–0.89) models. By contrast, no statistically significant association was evident under the dominant model (AA + AG vs. GG: OR = 0.78, 95%CI 0.54–1.12) (Figure 4).

Table 2. Characteristics of studies included in the meta-analysis.

Authors	Country	Study Design	Ethnicity	Sample Size	Sample	SNPs	Genotyping Method
Baczyńska-Strzecha et al., 2016 [9]	Poland	Case-control	Caucasian	199	Maternal blood	ApaI BsmI TaqI	TaqMan Assay
Javorski et al., 2018 [33]	Brazil	Case-control	Mixed	189	Maternal blood	FokI	TaqMan Assay
Rosenfeld et al., 2017 [34]	Israel	Case-control	Mixed	375	Maternal and fetal blood	ApaI BsmI FokI TaqI	RFLP
Mamma & Bambino Cohort, 2018	Italy	Prospective cohort	Caucasian	187	Maternal blood	ApaI BsmI FokI TaqI	TaqMan Assay

Abbreviations: SNP, single nucleotide polymorphism.

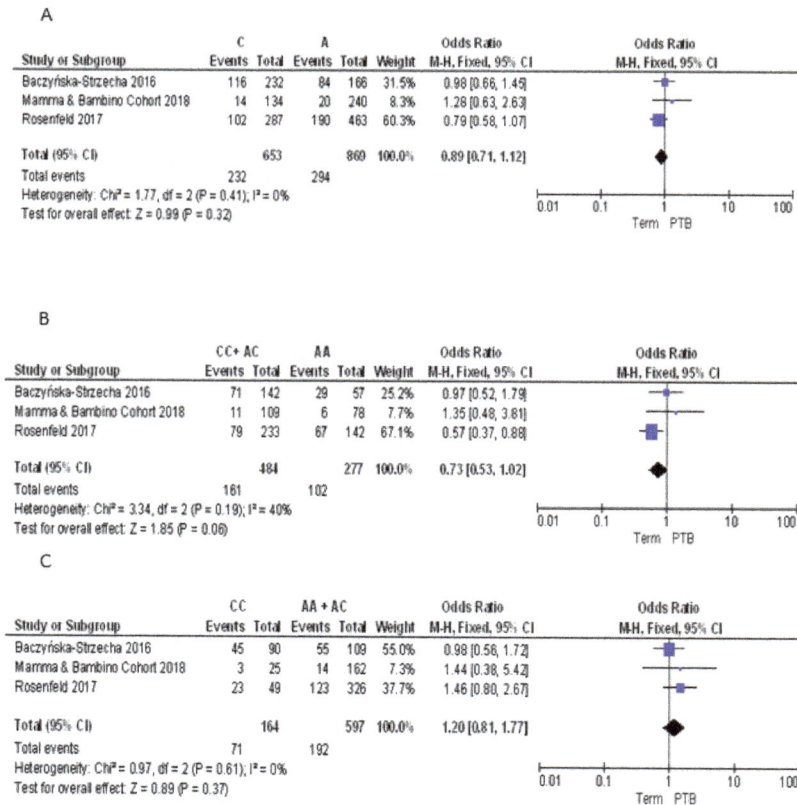

Figure 3. Forest plots of the association between ApaI polymorphism and preterm birth under the (**A**) allelic, (**B**) dominant and (**C**) recessive models.

For the FokI polymorphism we pooled our results with those reported by Javorski et al. and Rosenfeld et al. [33,34]. The Q-test and I^2 statistics showed significant heterogeneity across studies under the allelic ($p = 0.002$; $I^2 = 85\%$), dominant ($p = 0.02$; $I^2 = 74\%$) and recessive models ($p = 0.001$; $I^2 = 77\%$). Using the random effect model, the meta-analysis showed a significant association with PTB under the recessive model (AA vs. GG + AG: OR = 3.67, 95%CI 1.18–11.43). By contrast, pooled ORs under the allelic (A vs. G: OR = 1.90, 95%CI 0.96–3.75) and dominant (AA + AG vs. GG: OR = 1.65, 95%CI 0.80–3.42) models were not statistically significant (Figure 5).

A

Study or Subgroup	A Events	Total	G Events	Total	Weight	Odds Ratio M-H, Fixed, 95% CI
Baczyńska-Strzecha 2016	127	264	73	134	29.4%	0.77 [0.51, 1.18]
Mamma & Bambino Cohort 2018	14	138	20	236	7.8%	1.22 [0.59, 2.50]
Rosenfeld 2017	122	359	170	391	62.8%	0.67 [0.50, 0.90]
Total (95% CI)		761		761	100.0%	0.74 [0.59, 0.93]
Total events	263		263			

Heterogeneity: Chi² = 2.35, df = 2 (P = 0.31); I² = 15%
Test for overall effect: Z = 2.55 (P = 0.01)

B

Study or Subgroup	AA + AG Events	Total	GG Events	Total	Weight	Odds Ratio M-H, Fixed, 95% CI
Baczyńska-Strzecha 2016	86	172	14	27	18.7%	0.93 [0.41, 2.09]
Mamma & Bambino Cohort 2018	14	130	3	57	5.7%	2.17 [0.60, 7.88]
Rosenfeld 2017	90	254	56	121	75.6%	0.64 [0.41, 0.99]
Total (95% CI)		556		205	100.0%	0.78 [0.54, 1.12]
Total events	190		73			

Heterogeneity: Chi² = 3.42, df = 2 (P = 0.18); I² = 42%
Test for overall effect: Z = 1.34 (P = 0.18)

C

Study or Subgroup	AA Events	Total	AG + GG Events	Total	Weight	Odds Ratio M-H, Fixed, 95% CI
Baczyńska-Strzecha 2016	41	92	59	107	39.7%	0.65 [0.37, 1.15]
Mamma & Bambino Cohort 2018	0	8	17	179	2.1%	0.55 [0.03, 9.87]
Rosenfeld 2017	32	105	114	270	58.2%	0.60 [0.37, 0.97]
Total (95% CI)		205		556	100.0%	0.62 [0.43, 0.89]
Total events	73		190			

Heterogeneity: Chi² = 0.06, df = 2 (P = 0.97); I² = 0%
Test for overall effect: Z = 2.59 (P = 0.010)

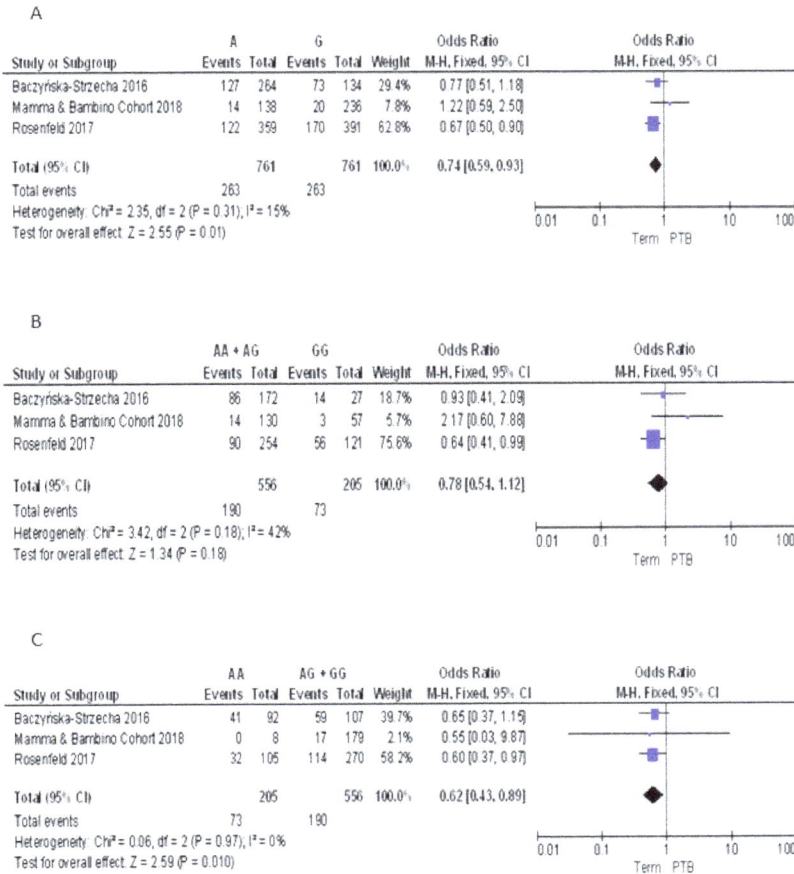

Figure 4. Forest plots of the association between BsmI polymorphism and preterm birth under the (**A**) allelic, (**B**) dominant and (**C**) recessive models.

A

Study or Subgroup	A Events	Total	G Events	Total	Weight	Odds Ratio M-H, Random, 95% CI
Javorski 2017	91	133	117	245	34.6%	2.37 [1.52, 3.69]
Mamma & Bambino Cohort 2018	18	108	16	266	28.0%	3.13 [1.53, 6.39]
Rosenfeld 2017	102	256	190	494	37.4%	1.06 [0.78, 1.44]
Total (95% CI)		497		1005	100.0%	1.90 [0.96, 3.75]
Total events	211		323			

Heterogeneity: Tau² = 0.30; Chi² = 12.99, df = 2 (P = 0.002); I² = 85%
Test for overall effect: Z = 1.84 (P = 0.07)

Odds Ratio M-H, Random, 95% CI (0.01 0.1 1 10 100 Term PTB)

B

Study or Subgroup	AA + AG Events	Total	GG Events	Total	Weight	Odds Ratio M-H, Random, 95% CI
Javorski 2017	67	105	37	84	36.1%	2.24 [1.25, 4.03]
Mamma & Bambino Cohort 2018	12	90	5	97	23.0%	2.83 [0.96, 8.39]
Rosenfeld 2017	79	207	67	168	40.8%	0.93 [0.61, 1.41]
Total (95% CI)		402		349	100.0%	1.65 [0.80, 3.42]
Total events	158		109			

Heterogeneity: Tau² = 0.29; Chi² = 7.71, df = 2 (P = 0.02); I² = 74%
Test for overall effect: Z = 1.35 (P = 0.18)

Odds Ratio M-H, Random, 95% CI (0.01 0.1 1 10 100 Term PTB)

C

Study or Subgroup	AA Events	Total	AG + GG Events	Total	Weight	Odds Ratio M-H, Random, 95% CI
Javorski 2017	24	28	80	161	31.0%	6.08 [2.02, 18.30]
Mamma & Bambino Cohort 2018	6	18	11	169	30.1%	7.18 [2.26, 22.79]
Rosenfeld 2017	23	49	123	326	38.9%	1.46 [0.80, 2.67]
Total (95% CI)		95		656	100.0%	3.67 [1.18, 11.43]
Total events	53		214			

Heterogeneity: Tau² = 0.77; Chi² = 8.74, df = 2 (P = 0.01); I² = 77%
Test for overall effect: Z = 2.24 (P = 0.02)

Odds Ratio M-H, Random, 95% CI (0.01 0.1 1 10 100 Term PTB)

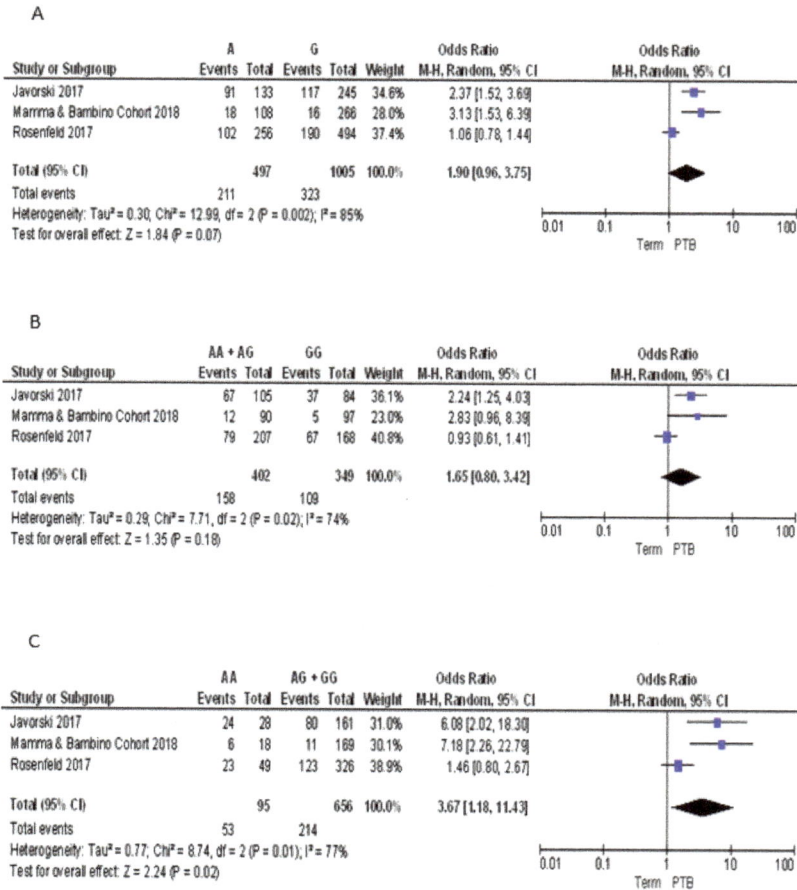

Figure 5. Forest plots of the association between FokI polymorphism and preterm birth under the (**A**) allelic, (**B**) dominant and (**C**) recessive models.

For the TaqI polymorphism we pooled our results with those reported by Baczyńska-Strzecha et al. and Rosenfeld et al. [9,34]. The Q-test and I^2 statistics showed no significant heterogeneity across studies under the allelic ($p = 0.29$; $I^2 = 19\%$), dominant ($p = 0.51$; $I^2 = 0\%$) and recessive ($p = 0.13$; $I^2 = 55\%$) models. Using the fixed effect model, the meta-analysis showed no significant association with PTB under the allelic (G vs. A: OR = 0.94, 95%CI 0.75–1.18), dominant (GG + AG vs. AA: OR = 0.88, 95%CI 0.63–1.21), and recessive (GG vs. AA + AG: OR = 1.00, 95%CI 0.69–1.46) models (Figure 6). Overall, we found no evidence of publication bias for meta-analyses of ApaI (Begg's $p = 0.74$; Egger's $p = 0.89$), BsmI (Begg's $p = 0.70$; Egger's $p = 0.19$), FokI (Begg's $p = 0.87$; Egger's $p = 0.81$), and TaqI (Begg's $p = 0.42$; Egger's $p = 0.24$).

A

B

C

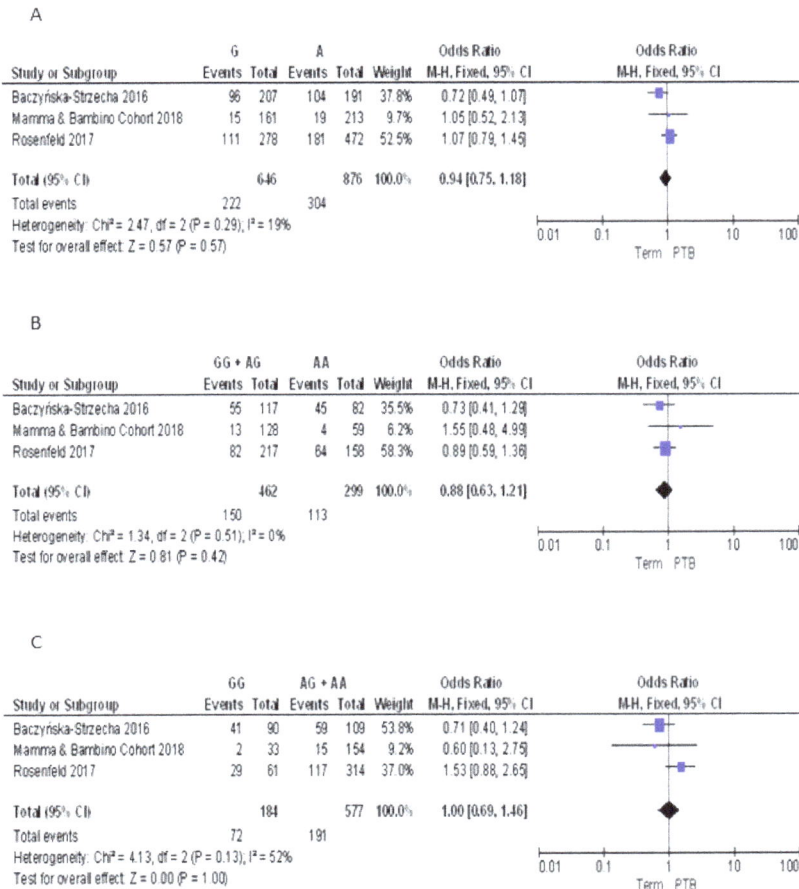

Figure 6. Forest plots of the association between TaqI polymorphism and preterm birth under the (**A**) allelic, (**B**) dominant and (**C**) recessive models.

4. Discussion

In the present study, we used data from the "Mamma & Bambino" cohort to evaluate the effect of VDR polymorphisms on neonatal anthropometric measures and on the risk of PTB. Interestingly, we observed that maternal FokI polymorphism affected both gestational duration and birth weight, which decreased with increased number of the mutated allele (A). This is consistent with Workalemahu and colleagues that demonstrated, for the first time, that birth weight decreased with increasing number of A allele [35]. In line with reduced gestational duration, we also demonstrated that the risk of PTB increased with increasing number of A allele both in the age-adjusted and in the multivariable-adjusted models. Notably, compared to mothers with GG or GA genotypes, mothers who carried the AA genotype exhibited a 12-fold increased risk of PTB, independent of socio-demographic characteristics (age, educational level, employment status), lifestyle (smoking, pre-gestational BMI, GWG), vitamin D intake, use of vitamin D supplements, type of delivery and parity. A similar risk was also observed by Manzon et al. [36] and Javorsky et al. [33], while Rosenfeld and colleagues failed in demonstrating this association. When we pooled our results with those reported by Javorsky et al. and Rosenfeld et al. [33,34], we demonstrated a significant positive association between FokI polymorphism and PTB under the recessive model. By contrast, Rosenfeld and colleagues [34] also demonstrated that the proportion of women with PTB decreased with increasing number of mutated allele (A) of maternal BsmI polymorphism. Although we failed in demonstrating this association, the meta-analysis confirmed the protective effect of BsmI against PTB under the allelic and recessive models. Results about the effect of TaqI polymorphism on PTB risk are currently inconclusive: while Manzon and colleagues proposed that the mutated allele conferred a lower PTB risk [36], we did not confirm this association by pooling our results with those reported by Baczyńska-Strzecha et al. and Rosenfeld et al. [9,34]. However, since we observed that birth weight increased with increasing number of mutated alleles, it cannot be completely excluded the protective effect of TaqI polymorphism on foetal growth and development. A prospective study on 615 pregnant women, conducted by Swamy and colleagues, evaluated the effect of 38 VDR polymorphisms on several birth outcomes. Since 8 of 38 SNPs examined—including ApaI—significantly affected birth weight in black but not in white women, the Authors concluded that strength of association may depend on ethnicity, proposing a partial explanation for the observed racial disparity in several pregnancy outcomes [37]. However, non-significant results in white women may be the result of the substantially smaller sample for compared to the black group. Nevertheless, comparison between studies should be interpreted with caution due to the high heterogeneity across studies in terms of design, sample size and type, ethnicity, geographical diversity, sun exposure, maternal habits and outcomes of interest, that may account for discrepancies in the obtained results [9,33,34].

The mechanistic link between VDR expression and foetal outcome is still unclear. Calcitriol is the major active ligand of VDR. The ligand-bound VDR forms a heterodimer with nuclear retinoid X receptor (RXR) [31], which recognizes vitamin D response elements (VDRE) in the promoter regions of vitamin D target genes and recruits co-factors to modulate gene transcription [32]. However, vitamin D can also exert rapid non-genomic effects, probably via VDR located within the plasma membrane [57]. This rapid pathway works via specific enzymes, such as protein kinase C and mitogen-activated protein kinase [57], which regulate cell proliferation and differentiation, invasive processes and apoptosis. Although several studies suggest that vitamin D system—including VDR, its ligands and the metabolizing enzymes—plays a key role in innate immunity and implantation [58–62], the functional effects of VDR and its allelic variants in pregnancy are not yet clarified. The main weakness of our study was the relatively small sample size and the statistical power—with a low number of PTB infants—that raises the need of future analyses on the ongoing "Mamma & Bambino" cohort to confirm the observed associations. Although we acknowledge that further stratification by ethnicity should be provided—the "Mamma & Bambino" cohort consisted of Caucasian women—we established the effect of VDR polymorphisms on PTB risk in the context of previous studies investigating this association in medium-large populations that included different racial and ethnic groups. However, due to inconsistency of reported outcomes, we cannot perform a meta-analysis of the association between VDR polymorphisms and neonatal anthropometric measures. Indeed, only three studies investigated the effect on neonatal anthropometric measures using birth weight [37], LBW [35] or SGA [41] as primary outcome. Furthermore, the collection of additional data regarding other anthropometric measures should be included in future studies. Another weakness was that we did not analysed VDR polymorphisms in infant samples, not being able to assess the contribution of foetal VDR gene on adverse pregnancy outcomes. In fact, as reported by Rosenfeld et al., the risk of PTB could be higher in new-borns carrying the non-mutated BsmI or the mutated ApaI allele [34]. Moreover, the influence of unmeasured variables, such as sun exposure, maternal habits and serum vitamin D levels cannot be completely excluded. Since the FFQ did not quantify vitamin D from nutritional supplements and fortified foods, we did not have a precise measure of vitamin D intake status. However, we reported that the use of vitamin D supplements containing is not common among women from the "Mamma % Bambino" cohort and no association with PTB risk was evident. Furthermore, the measurement of 25OHD would be useful to evaluate whether there was a relationship between serum levels and dietary intake, including vitamin D supplements. In addition, it should be recognized that, in the present

Nutrients **2018**, *10*, 1172

study, other variables such as poverty status, mid-pregnancy immune and growth-related factors, recently associated with PTB prediction in women with and without preeclampsia [63], have not been included. Notably, our study was conducted in a cohort of the women in Sicily, southern Italy and a recent systematic review reports that despite high levels of sunshine, maternal hypovitaminosis D during pregnancy is prevalent in sunny Mediterranean region where optimal vitamin D levels are expected [64]. Reasons for this phenomenon may rely on different factors that can determine vitamin D deficiency.

Finally, in future studies the effects of other single nucleotide polymorphisms in genes encoding for key components of the vitamin D metabolism pathway—such as genes involved in cholesterol synthesis (DHCR7), hydroxylation (CYP2R1, CYP24A1), and vitamin D transport (GC) that influence vitamin D status [64,65] should be addressed. We acknowledge that unmeasured variables in the current analysis limit our ability to draw conclusions on the association of maternal VDR polymorphisms with neonatal anthropometric measures and the risk of PTB in our cohort. Despite such limitations, the strictly selection criteria ruled out potential confounders such as pre-existing medical conditions, pregnancy complications, pre-term induced delivery or caesarean section, intrauterine foetal death, plurality and congenital malformations. Moreover, extensive data collection enabled to adjust our results for socio-demographic factors, lifestyle, pre-gestational BMI and GWG, and vitamin D dietary intake. Additional researches, including observational prospective studies and clinical trials, are recommended to establish the role of vitamin D and related factors in pregnancy, and to develop and validate effective preventive strategies against adverse outcomes.

5. Conclusions

In conclusion, we provide novel evidence and a meta-analysis about the effect of VDR polymorphisms on birth weight and gestational duration, identifying a group of women at risk of PTB.

Author Contributions: Conceptualization, M.B., A.M. and A.A.; Methodology, M.B., A.M. and A.A.; Formal Analysis, A.M., R.M.S.L. and G.F.; Data Curation, A.M., M.C.L.R., R.M.S.L. and G.F.; Writing-Original Draft Preparation, M.B., A.M., R.M.S.L., G.F. and A.A.; Writing-Review & Editing, all the Authors; Supervision, M.B. and A.A.; Project Administration, M.B., M.P., A.C. and A.A.; Funding Acquisition, A.A.

Funding: This research was funded by the Department of Medical and Surgical Sciences and Advanced Technologies "GF Ingrassia", University of Catania, Italy (*Piano Triennale di Sviluppo delle Attività di Ricerca Scientifica del Dipartimento 2016–18*).

Conflicts of Interest: The authors declare no conflict of interest.

References

1. Chiavaroli, V.; Castorani, V.; Guidone, P.; Derraik, J.G.; Liberati, M.; Chiarelli, F.; Mohn, A. Incidence of infants born small- and large-for-gestational-age in an italian cohort over a 20-year period and associated risk factors. *Ital. J. Pediatr.* **2016**, *42*, 42. [CrossRef] [PubMed]
2. Lawn, J.E.; Blencowe, H.; Pattinson, R.; Cousens, S.; Kumar, R.; Ibiebele, I.; Gardosi, J.; Day, L.T.; Stanton, C. Stillbirths: Where? When? Why? How to make the data count? *Lancet* **2011**, *377*, 1448–1463. [CrossRef]
3. Goldenberg, R.L.; Culhane, J.F.; Iams, J.D.; Romero, R. Epidemiology and causes of preterm birth. *Lancet* **2008**, *371*, 75–84. [CrossRef]
4. Howson, C.P.; Kinney, M.V.; McDougall, L.; Lawn, J.E. Born too soon: Preterm birth matters. *Reprod. Health* **2013**, *10* (Suppl. 1), S1. [CrossRef] [PubMed]
5. Vogel, J.P.; Chawanpaiboon, S.; Moller, A.B.; Watananirun, K.; Bonet, M.; Lumbiganon, P. The global epidemiology of preterm birth. *Best Pract. Res. Clin. Obstet. Gynaecol.* **2018**, in press. [CrossRef] [PubMed]
6. Vitale, S.G.; Marilli, I.; Rapisarda, A.M.; Rossetti, D.; Belluomo, G.; Iapichino, V.; Stancanelli, F.; Cianci, A. Cellular and biochemical mechanisms, risk factors and management of preterm birth: State of the art. *Minerva Ginecol.* **2014**, *66*, 589–595. [PubMed]
7. Giunta, G.; Giuffrida, L.; Mangano, K.; Fagone, P.; Cianci, A. Influence of lactoferrin in preventing preterm delivery: A pilot study. *Mol. Med. Rep.* **2012**, *5*, 162–166. [PubMed]

8.   Pino, A.; Giunta, G.; Randazzo, C.L.; Caruso, S.; Caggia, C.; Cianci, A. Bacterial biota of women with bacterial vaginosis treated with lactoferrin: An open prospective randomized trial. *Microb. Ecol. Health Dis.* **2017**, *28*, 1357417. [CrossRef] [PubMed]

9.   Baczyńska-Strzecha, M.; Kalinka, J. Influence of apa1 (rs7975232), taq1 (rs731236) and bsm1 (rs154410) polymorphisms of vitamin d receptor on preterm birth risk in the polish population. *Ginekol. Pol.* **2016**, *87*, 763–768. [CrossRef] [PubMed]

10. York, T.P.; Eaves, L.J.; Neale, M.C.; Strauss, J.F. The contribution of genetic and environmental factors to the duration of pregnancy. *Am. J. Obstet. Gynecol.* **2014**, *210*, 398–405. [CrossRef] [PubMed]

11. Black, R.E. Global prevalence of small for gestational age births. *Nestle Nutr. Inst. Workshop Ser.* **2015**, *81*, 1–7. [PubMed]

12. Chavarro, J.E.; Rich-Edwards, J.W.; Rosner, B.A.; Willett, W.C. Iron intake and risk of ovulatory infertility. *Obstet. Gynecol.* **2006**, *108*, 1145–1152. [CrossRef] [PubMed]

13. Lieberman, E.; Gremy, I.; Lang, J.M.; Cohen, A.P. Low birthweight at term and the timing of fetal exposure to maternal smoking. *Am. J. Public Health* **1994**, *84*, 1127–1131. [CrossRef] [PubMed]

14. Pietrantoni, M.; Knuppel, R.A. Alcohol use in pregnancy. *Clin. Perinatol.* **1991**, *18*, 93–111. [CrossRef]

15. Fowles, E.R. Prenatal nutrition and birth outcomes. *J. Obstet. Gynecol. Neonatal. Nurs.* **2004**, *33*, 809–822. [CrossRef] [PubMed]

16. Ji, J.L.; Muyayalo, K.P.; Zhang, Y.H.; Hu, X.H.; Liao, A.H. Immunological function of vitamin D during human pregnancy. *Am. J. Reprod. Immunol.* **2017**, *78*. [CrossRef] [PubMed]

17. Kiely, M.; Hemmingway, A.; O'Callaghan, K.M. Vitamin D in pregnancy: Current perspectives and future directions. *Ther. Adv. Musculoskelet. Dis.* **2017**, *9*, 145–154. [CrossRef] [PubMed]

18. Holick, M.F. Vitamin D: A D-lightful solution for health. *J. Investig. Med.* **2011**, *59*, 872–880. [CrossRef] [PubMed]

19. Institute of Medicine. *Dietary Reference Intakes for Calcium and Vitamin D*; The National Academies Press: Washington, DC, USA, 2011.

20. U.S. Department of Agriculture, Agricultural Research Service (ARS). USDA National Nutrient Database for Standard Reference. Available online: https://www.ars.usda.gov/northeast-area/beltsville-md-bhnrc/beltsville-human-nutrition-research-center/nutrient-data-laboratory/docs/usda-national-nutrient-database-for-standard-reference/ (accessed on 1 May 2018).

21. Ovesen, L.; Brot, C.; Jakobsen, J. Food contents and biological activity of 25-hydroxyvitamin D: A vitamin D metabolite to be reckoned with? *Ann. Nutr. Metab.* **2003**, *47*, 107–113. [CrossRef] [PubMed]

22. Calvo, M.S.; Whiting, S.J.; Barton, C.N. Vitamin D fortification in the United States and Canada: Current status and data needs. *Am. J. Clin. Nutr.* **2004**, *80*, 1710S–1716S. [CrossRef] [PubMed]

23. Holick, M.F. Vitamin D: A millenium perspective. *J. Cell. Biochem.* **2003**, *88*, 296–307. [CrossRef] [PubMed]

24. Norman, A.W. The history of the discovery of vitamin D and its daughter steroid hormone. *Ann. Nutr. Metab.* **2012**, *61*, 199–206. [CrossRef] [PubMed]

25. Harvey, N.C.; Holroyd, C.; Ntani, G.; Javaid, K.; Cooper, P.; Moon, R.; Cole, Z.; Tinati, T.; Godfrey, K.; Dennison, E.; et al. Vitamin D supplementation in pregnancy: A systematic review. *Health Technol. Assess.* **2014**, *18*, 1–190. [CrossRef] [PubMed]

26. De-Regil, L.M.; Palacios, C.; Lombardo, L.K.; Peña-Rosas, J.P. Vitamin D supplementation for women during pregnancy. *Sao Paulo Med. J.* **2016**, *134*, 274–275. [CrossRef] [PubMed]

27. Pérez-López, F.R.; Pasupuleti, V.; Mezones-Holguin, E.; Benites-Zapata, V.A.; Thota, P.; Deshpande, A.; Hernandez, A.V. Effect of vitamin D supplementation during pregnancy on maternal and neonatal outcomes: A systematic review and meta-analysis of randomized controlled trials. *Fertil. Steril.* **2015**, *103*, 1278–1288.e4. [CrossRef] [PubMed]

28. Thorne-Lyman, A.; Fawzi, W.W. Vitamin D during pregnancy and maternal, neonatal and infant health outcomes: A systematic review and meta-analysis. *Paediatr. Perinat. Epidemiol.* **2012**, *26* (Suppl. 1), 75–90. [CrossRef] [PubMed]

29. Strugnell, S.A.; Deluca, H.F. The vitamin d receptor-structure and transcriptional activation. *Proc. Soc. Exp. Biol. Med.* **1997**, *215*, 223–228. [CrossRef] [PubMed]

30. Wang, Y.; Zhu, J.; DeLuca, H.F. Where is the vitamin D receptor? *Arch. Biochem. Biophys.* **2012**, *523*, 123–133. [CrossRef] [PubMed]

31. Freedman, L.P.; Arce, V.; Perez Fernandez, R. DNA sequences that act as high affinity targets for the vitamin D3 receptor in the absence of the retinoid x receptor. *Mol. Endocrinol.* **1994**, *8*, 265–273. [PubMed]

32. Karras, S.N.; Wagner, C.L.; Castracane, V.D. Understanding vitamin d metabolism in pregnancy: From physiology to pathophysiology and clinical outcomes. *Metabolism* **2018**, *86*, 112–123. [CrossRef] [PubMed]

33. Javorski, N.; Lima, C.A.D.; Silva, L.V.C.; Crovella, S.; de Azêvedo Silva, J. Vitamin D receptor (VDR) polymorphisms are associated to spontaneous preterm birth and maternal aspects. *Gene* **2018**, *642*, 58–63. [CrossRef] [PubMed]

34. Rosenfeld, T.; Salem, H.; Altarescu, G.; Grisaru-Granovsky, S.; Tevet, A.; Birk, R. Maternal-fetal vitamin D receptor polymorphisms significantly associated with preterm birth. *Arch. Gynecol. Obstet.* **2017**, *296*, 215–222. [CrossRef] [PubMed]

35. Workalemahu, T.; Badon, S.E.; Dishi-Galitzky, M.; Qiu, C.; Williams, M.A.; Sorensen, T.; Enquobahrie, D.A. Placental genetic variations in vitamin D metabolism and birthweight. *Placenta* **2017**, *50*, 78–83. [CrossRef] [PubMed]

36. Manzon, L.; Altarescu, G.; Tevet, A.; Schimmel, M.S.; Elstein, D.; Samueloff, A.; Grisaru-Granovsky, S. Vitamin D receptor polymorphism foki is associated with spontaneous idiopathic preterm birth in an israeli population. *Eur. J. Obstet. Gynecol. Reprod. Biol.* **2014**, *177*, 84–88. [CrossRef] [PubMed]

37. Swamy, G.K.; Garrett, M.E.; Miranda, M.L.; Ashley-Koch, A.E. Maternal vitamin D receptor genetic variation contributes to infant birthweight among black mothers. *Am. J. Med. Genet. A* **2011**, *155A*, 1264–1271. [CrossRef] [PubMed]

38. Lorentzon, M.; Lorentzon, R.; Nordström, P. Vitamin D receptor gene polymorphism is associated with birth height, growth to adolescence, and adult stature in healthy Caucasian men: A cross-sectional and longitudinal study. *J. Clin. Endocrinol. Metab.* **2000**, *85*, 1666–1670. [PubMed]

39. Tao, C.; Yu, T.; Garnett, S.; Briody, J.; Knight, J.; Woodhead, H.; Cowell, C.T. Vitamin D receptor alleles predict growth and bone density in girls. *Arch. Dis. Child.* **1998**, *79*, 488–494. [CrossRef] [PubMed]

40. Suarez, F.; Zeghoud, F.; Rossignol, C.; Walrant, O.; Garabédian, M. Association between vitamin d receptor gene polymorphism and sex-dependent growth during the first two years of life. *J. Clin. Endocrinol. Metab.* **1997**, *82*, 2966–2970. [CrossRef] [PubMed]

41. Silvano, L.; Miras, M.; Pérez, A.; Picotto, G.; Díaz de Barboza, G.; Muñoz, L.; Martin, S.; Sobrero, G.; Armelini, P.; Mericq, V.; et al. Comparative analysis of clinical, biochemical and genetic aspects associated with bone mineral density in small for gestational age children. *J. Pediatr. Endocrinol. Metab.* **2011**, *24*, 511–517. [CrossRef] [PubMed]

42. Suarez, F.; Rossignol, C.; Garabédian, M. Interactive effect of estradiol and vitamin D receptor gene polymorphisms as a possible determinant of growth in male and female infants. *J. Clin. Endocrinol. Metab.* **1998**, *83*, 3563–3568. [CrossRef] [PubMed]

43. Knabl, J.; Vattai, A.; Ye, Y.; Jueckstock, J.; Hutter, S.; Kainer, F.; Mahner, S.; Jeschke, U. Role of placental VDR expression and function in common late pregnancy disorders. *Int. J. Mol. Sci.* **2017**, *18*, E2340. [CrossRef] [PubMed]

44. Agodi, A.; Barchitta, M.; Quattrocchi, A.; Maugeri, A.; Vinciguerra, M. Dapk1 promoter methylation and cervical cancer risk: A systematic review and a meta-analysis. *PLoS ONE* **2015**, *10*, e0135078. [CrossRef] [PubMed]

45. Agodi, A.; Barchitta, M.; Quattrocchi, A.; Maugeri, A.; Canto, C.; Marchese, A.E.; Vinciguerra, M. Low fruit consumption and folate deficiency are associated with line-1 hypomethylation in women of a cancer-free population. *Genes Nutr.* **2015**, *10*, 480. [CrossRef] [PubMed]

46. Barchitta, M.; Quattrocchi, A.; Maugeri, A.; Vinciguerra, M.; Agodi, A. Line-1 hypomethylation in blood and tissue samples as an epigenetic marker for cancer risk: A systematic review and meta-analysis. *PLoS ONE* **2014**, *9*, e109478. [CrossRef] [PubMed]

47. Barchitta, M.; Quattrocchi, A.; Maugeri, A.; Canto, C.; La Rosa, N.; Cantarella, M.A.; Spampinato, G.; Scalisi, A.; Agodi, A. Line-1 hypermethylation in white blood cell dna is associated with high-grade cervical intraepithelial neoplasia. *BMC Cancer* **2017**, *17*, 601. [CrossRef] [PubMed]

48. Barchitta, M.; Maugeri, A.; Quattrocchi, A.; Agrifoglio, O.; Agodi, A. The role of mirnas as biomarkers for pregnancy outcomes: A comprehensive review. *Int. J. Genomics* **2017**, *2017*, 8067972. [CrossRef] [PubMed]

49. Physical status: The use and interpretation of anthropometry: Report of a WHO expert committee. *World Health Organ. Tech. Rep. Ser.* **1995**, *854*, 1–452.

50. Moore Simas, T.A.; Waring, M.E.; Sullivan, G.M.; Liao, X.; Rosal, M.C.; Hardy, J.R.; Berry, R.E. Institute of medicine 2009 gestational weight gain guideline knowledge: Survey of obstetrics/gynecology and family medicine residents of the united states. *Birth* **2013**, *40*, 237–246. [CrossRef] [PubMed]

51. Bertino, E.; Spada, E.; Occhi, L.; Coscia, A.; Giuliani, F.; Gagliardi, L.; Gilli, G.; Bona, G.; Fabris, C.; De Curtis, M.; et al. Neonatal anthropometric charts: The Italian neonatal study compared with other European studies. *J. Pediatr. Gastroenterol. Nutr.* **2010**, *51*, 353–361. [CrossRef] [PubMed]

52. Agodi, A.; Barchitta, M.; Valenti, G.; Marzagalli, R.; Frontini, V.; Marchese, A.E. Increase in the prevalence of the mthfr 677 tt polymorphism in women born since 1959: Potential implications for folate requirements. *Eur. J. Clin. Nutr.* **2011**, *65*, 1302–1308. [CrossRef] [PubMed]

53. Higgins, J.P.; Thompson, S.G. Quantifying heterogeneity in a meta-analysis. *Stat. Med.* **2002**, *21*, 1539–1558. [CrossRef] [PubMed]

54. Higgins, J.P.; Green, S. Cochrane Handbook for Systematic Reviews of Interventions, Version 5.1.0 ed. 2008. Available online: https://handbook-5-1.cochrane.org/ (accessed on 1 March 2018).

55. Begg, C.B.; Mazumdar, M. Operating characteristics of a rank correlation test for publication bias. *Biometrics* **1994**, *50*, 1088–1101. [CrossRef] [PubMed]

56. Egger, M.; Davey Smith, G.; Schneider, M.; Minder, C. Bias in meta-analysis detected by a simple, graphical test. *BMJ* **1997**, *315*, 629–634. [CrossRef] [PubMed]

57. Shin, J.S.; Choi, M.Y.; Longtine, M.S.; Nelson, D.M. Vitamin D effects on pregnancy and the placenta. *Placenta* **2010**, *31*, 1027–1034. [CrossRef] [PubMed]

58. Evans, K.N.; Bulmer, J.N.; Kilby, M.D.; Hewison, M. Vitamin D and placental-decidual function. *J. Soc. Gynecol. Investig.* **2004**, *11*, 263–271. [CrossRef] [PubMed]

59. Stephanou, A.; Ross, R.; Handwerger, S. Regulation of human placental lactogen expression by 1,25-dihydroxyvitamin d3. *Endocrinology* **1994**, *135*, 2651–2656. [CrossRef] [PubMed]

60. Avila, E.; Díaz, L.; Barrera, D.; Halhali, A.; Méndez, I.; González, L.; Zuegel, U.; Steinmeyer, A.; Larrea, F. Regulation of vitamin D hydroxylases gene expression by 1,25-dihydroxyvitamin d3 and cyclic amp in cultured human syncytiotrophoblasts. *J. Steroid. Biochem. Mol. Biol.* **2007**, *103*, 90–96. [CrossRef] [PubMed]

61. Evans, K.N.; Nguyen, L.; Chan, J.; Innes, B.A.; Bulmer, J.N.; Kilby, M.D.; Hewison, M. Effects of 25-hydroxyvitamin d3 and 1,25-dihydroxyvitamin d3 on cytokine production by human decidual cells. *Biol. Reprod.* **2006**, *75*, 816–822. [CrossRef] [PubMed]

62. Murthi, P.; Yong, H.E.; Ngyuen, T.P.; Ellery, S.; Singh, H.; Rahman, R.; Dickinson, H.; Walker, D.W.; Davies-Tuck, M.; Wallace, E.M.; et al. Role of the placental vitamin d receptor in modulating feto-placental growth in fetal growth restriction and preeclampsia-affected pregnancies. *Front. Physiol.* **2016**, *7*, 43. [CrossRef] [PubMed]

63. Jelliffe-Pawlowski, L.L.; Rand, L.; Bedell, B.; Baer, R.J.; Oltman, S.P.; Norton, M.E.; Shaw, G.M.; Stevenson, D.K.; Murray, J.C.; Ryckman, K.K. Correction: Prediction of preterm birth with and without preeclampsia using mid-pregnancy immune and growth-related molecular factors and maternal characteristics. *J. Perinatol.* **2018**, *38*, 946. [CrossRef] [PubMed]

64. Karras, S.; Paschou, S.A.; Kandaraki, E.; Anagnostis, P.; Annweiler, C.; Tarlatzis, B.C.; Hollis, B.W.; Grant, W.B.; Goulis, D.G. Hypovitaminosis D in pregnancy in the Mediterranean region: A systematic review. *Eur. J. Clin. Nutr.* **2016**, *70*, 979–986. [CrossRef] [PubMed]

65. Wang, T.J.; Zhang, F.; Richards, J.B.; Kestenbaum, B.; van Meurs, J.B.; Berry, D.; Kiel, D.P.; Streeten, E.A.; Ohlsson, C.; Koller, D.L.; et al. Common genetic determinants of vitamin d insufficiency: A genome-wide association study. *Lancet* **2010**, *376*, 180–188. [CrossRef]

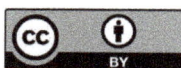

![nutrients logo] *nutrients*

MDPI

Article

Compliance to Prenatal Iron and Folic Acid Supplement Use in Relation to Low Birth Weight in Lilongwe, Malawi

Aaron Thokozani Chikakuda [1,†], Dayeon Shin [2], Sarah S. Comstock [1], SuJin Song [3,‡] and Won O. Song [1,*]

1   Department of Food Science and Human Nutrition, Michigan State University, East Lansing, MI 48824, USA; achikakuda@luanar.ac.mw (A.T.C.); comsto37@msu.edu (S.S.C.)
2   Department of Public Health, Food Studies and Nutrition, Syracuse University, Syracuse, NY 13244, USA; dshin03@syr.edu
3   Department of Food and Nutrition, Hannam University, Daejeon 34054, Korea; sjsong@hnu.kr
*   Correspondence: song@msu.edu; Tel.: +1-517-353-3332
†   Current address: Department of Human Nutrition and Health, Lilongwe University of Agriculture & Natural Resources (LUANAR), P.O. Box 219 Lilongwe, Malawi.
‡   S.S. was a post-doctoral fellow in the research team at the time when the research was carried out.

Received: 5 July 2018; Accepted: 6 September 2018; Published: 10 September 2018

check for updates

Abstract: Prenatal iron and folic acid (IFA) supplements are offered free to all pregnant women in Malawi to reduce maternal anemia and improve birth outcomes. We investigated the association between self-reported compliance to IFA intake and risk of low birth weight (LBW). Pregnant women who attended Bwaila Maternity Wing of Lilongwe District Hospital for delivery were recruited (n = 220). We used a questionnaire to collect self-reported information on IFA use and maternal sociodemographic data. Before delivery, blood samples for maternal hemoglobin (Hb) and folate status, and upon delivery, birth weight, and other newborn anthropometrics were measured. We used multivariable logistic regression to determine risk of LBW by prenatal IFA intake. The self-reported number of IFA pills taken during pregnancy was positively associated with Hb, but not serum and RBC folate concentration: <45, 45–89 and ≥90 pills taken corresponded with mean (SD) Hb 10.7 (1.6), 11.3 (1.8), and 11.7 (1.6) g/dL, respectively (p = 0.006). The prevalence of LBW was 20.1%, 13.5% and 5.6% for those who reported taking IFA pills <45, 45–89, and ≥90 pills, respectively (p = 0.027). Taking >60 IFA pills reduced risk of LBW delivery (OR (95% CI) = 0.15 (0.03–0.70), p = 0.033) than taking ≤30 pills. Self-reported compliance to IFA use is valid for assessing prenatal supplement program in Malawi, especially Hb status, and can reduce the rate of LBW.

Keywords: prenatal iron and folic acid (IFA) supplements; low birth weight; maternal anemia; Malawi

1. Introduction

Low birth weight (LBW) is internationally recognized as a birth weight below 2500 g (5.5 pounds). LBW is a birth outcome of importance to public health, associated with increased morbidity and mortality in neonates and infants and cardiovascular disease risks later in life [1–3]. This practical cutoff for international comparison is based on epidemiological observations that LBW babies are 20 times more likely to die than heavier infants [4].

Over 20 million infants worldwide are born with LBW. More than half of LBW babies are born in developing countries, particularly South-Central Asia, where more than 27% of the babies born weigh less than 2500 g. LBW prevalence in Sub-Saharan Africa (15%) is similar to the level in the Caribbean region (14%). The Central America and Oceania region has a LBW rate of about 10% [4]. LBW is still a leading cause of neonatal and infant mortality in the U.S. and other industrialized countries, although this prevalence is still much lower than that in developing countries [5].

More than half of LBW babies are born in developing countries and Malawi is as affected as other developing countries, with a LBW prevalence of above-the-world average. The national prevalence of LBW in Malawi is 12%, with the highest prevalence seen among mothers younger than 20 years of age (16%) and those older than 35 years of age. The Central region has a higher prevalence of LBW than Northern and Southern regions within Malawi [6].

Micronutrient deficiencies during pregnancy, particularly iron and folate, contribute significantly to the prevalence of LBW [7]. In a recently reported study in China, correction of micronutrient deficiency in pregnancy with prenatal supplementation improved birth outcomes [8]. LBW contributes significantly to neonatal and infant morbidity and mortality in Malawi. Despite the Malawian government's efforts to improve birth outcomes and health status for Malawians, the prevalence of most health risk indicators remains high. Anemia prevalence has gone up in reproductive age and pregnant women from 28 to 33% and 38 to 45%, from 2010 to 2016, respectively. The current maternal mortality rate of 497/100,000 live births indicates the need to improve maternal and child health. Maternal and infant mortality indicates the level of quality of healthcare available to citizens in a country [9]. For example, a high maternal mortality rate might be from high anemia that negatively affects birth outcomes and health of newborns [10,11]. This might indicate that there are inadequate screening and treatment services available for pregnant women, as evidenced by the high anemia prevalent in reproductive age women and pregnant women in Malawi. The nutritional status of children is poor, as indicated by 37% of children under the age of five being stunted [6].

Micronutrient supplements improve maternal nutrition status and birth outcomes [12–15]. The Generation R study in Rotterdam, the Netherlands, found that folic acid supplements increased weight at birth by 68 g and placental weight by 13 g in the supplemented group higher than those not supplemented [16]. In another study in northern China, multiple micronutrient supplements, which included IFA, increased birth weight, especially in those who had a low hemoglobin status at baseline [8]. Anemia is one of the biggest contributors of low birth [7,17]. In a case control study in Sudan, antenatal hemoglobin status was found to have modulating effects on birth outcomes, particularly LBW [7].

There have been clinical studies showing the efficacy of supplements in increasing biomarker status. However, these were conducted in controlled environments, while in real life people take medications freely at home. There have been no studies in Malawi showing how self-reported use of prenatal supplements increases hemoglobin and folate status. This in turn will validate self-reported intake of prenatal supplements as a reliable compliance monitoring method, which can be used to predict birth outcomes. We thus hypothesized that the self-reported number of IFA taken during pregnancy is inversely associated with LBW risks mediated by increased levels of maternal hemoglobin.

2. Materials and Methods

2.1. Study Subjects

The retrospective cross-sectional study design was not pre-specified and was considered exploratory. All pregnant women reporting for delivery at the Bwaila Maternity Wing of Lilongwe District Hospital were asked to participate in the study. Recruitment of subjects followed convenience sampling and included women of all age groups with viable singleton pregnancy or twin gestation delivering at 28 weeks or more. The women resided in Lilongwe district (rural, peri-urban or urban), which is the catchment area for this hospital. We recruited women with pregnancies of various gestation ages (28 weeks and upwards).

The study excluded dyads where the mother had severe anemia (requiring a blood transfusion), the presence of placenta previa (or history of bleeding during pregnancy due to early partial separation of placenta), delivery involved instrumentation, and those where an infant had brain trauma.

Additionally, participants must not have had a severe medical condition known to severely affect maternal nutrition status, placenta health, or newborn health. In summary, we excluded all obstetrical and medical emergencies. Babies and mothers that were in intensive care unit (ICU), high dependence unit (HDU), or required constant medical support and monitoring were excluded, so that their medical care was not interrupted. Of the 220 pregnant women who consented to participating in the study, seven who delivered twins were excluded from the final analysis. The final analytic sample size included 213 pregnant women.

2.2. Ethical Clearance/Institutional Review Board Approval

Ethical clearance or institutional review board approval was obtained from Michigan State University and the National Health Sciences Research Committee (NHSRC) in Malawi. At the hospital level, the Lilongwe District Health Officer (DHO), the overseer of all health services in the district, was contacted for approval to use the facility and their patients, and a letter of support for this research was issued. The nurse/midwife in-charge of the maternity unit was contacted for support. She informed the members of the staff in the unit about the study and urged them to offer daily support to the data collection. We obtained consent from the pregnant women or their mother/husband. If a woman was unable to write, we obtained a fingerprint of her thumb of non-dominant hand as a proof of her consent to voluntarily participate in the research study. Data and blood sample collection only commenced after the women gave voluntary consent to participate in the study.

2.3. IFA Pills

The Malawian government uses prenatal supplements as a short-term solution to fight micronutrient malnutrition (particularly iron deficiency anemia) in pregnant women and improve the health status of mothers and newborns. All pregnant women, regardless of hematological status or the trimester of pregnancy, receive prenatal supplements of pills of combined iron and folic acid from the first antenatal care visit to delivery. Each tablet contains 60 mg iron (ferrous) and 0.25 mg folic acid, taken once a day. Every month, the woman gets a new supply without a check if she actually utilized the prescription given the previous month. The program is run on the assumption that women understand the need to take the supplements, despite documented evidence of poor compliance due to side effects and women forgetting to take the pills [18,19]. Monitoring prenatal supplementation intake has been continued because it is the most feasible way to fight micronutrient malnutrition and improve health outcomes at least in the short term, compared to diet, considering the current social economic status of Malawians.

2.4. Demographics, Antenatal Care, and Maternal Anthropometrics

Using a short questionnaire, the basic characteristics of the pregnant woman were collected: age of the mother, gestation age, gravidity (number of pregnancies), parity (number of deliveries), education level of the mother, and area of residence.

The questionnaire also contained questions on antenatal care that the pregnant woman was able to access during pregnancy. This included information on IFA supplement use, which was obtained from self-reports and confirmed by checking medical records (health passport book, a little handbook that contains all medical information and previous treatments; the women carry the book everywhere). We used the same questions as those used in the Malawi demographic and health survey [6]. The questions ask if the participant received or bought IFA supplements in pregnancy; if she took any of the IFA pills; how many pills she was able to take during pregnancy. Our questionnaire also included questions on the number of antenatal visits the woman received, at what gestation of the pregnancy (trimester) did she start prenatal care, and reasons for starting prenatal care early or late [19]. Information about vaccinations, malaria prophylaxis, and use of anti-helminthes (anti-worms) during pregnancy was abstracted from the medical record (health passport book). We also obtained medical history about sickness during the current pregnancy, such as anemia (blood transfusions) and if the pregnant woman was on any long-term treatment or chronic diseases such as diabetes, hypertension and asthma/allergies. History of contraceptive use prior to the current pregnancy was obtained [20,21].

Maternal weight was taken on the day of the survey just before delivery of the baby using Seca weighing scale (Seca, Chino, CA, USA). Weight was measured to the nearest 0.1 kg in mothers. The midwives performed the anthropometric measurements on pregnant women who participated in the study. The women's height was measured using a stadiometer. They had to remove anything that she was wearing on her head and ensure that her braided hair was as flat as possible by loosening her hair and pressing her headpiece. The women also had to remove their shoes and heavy clothing (subjects were dressed in light clothes) during the anthropometric measurement process. Height was recorded to the nearest 0.1 cm. Most of the maternal characteristics are routinely documented on the labor-monitoring chart; therefore, only the parameters that are not available from the chart were asked to avoid duplication.

2.5. Blood Specimen Collection

We collected blood samples from women before they gave birth. Upon obtaining consent and explaining the procedure, the women was asked to sit or lie on a bed, as per their preference. A tourniquet was applied around the upper left arm and a 70% alcohol swab was used to clean the skin on the site (cubital). A 10 mL syringe with 21-gauge needle (SkyRun Pharma Co., Ltd., Nanjing, China) was then used to withdraw a venous whole blood sample from the cubital region.

Each blood specimen was collected in two different sample tubes of 5 mL each—one for serum and the other for red blood cell (RBC) folate analysis. The third specimen type was taken using a Microcuvette from the same 10 mL to measure iron status (hemoglobin). The blood sample for folate was allowed to flow freely into the specimen bottle by vacuum pressure, after piercing the rubber cover with the needle of the syringe.

The sample for RBC folate analysis was put in a 5 mL tube containing an anticoagulant (ethylenediaminetetraacetic acid, EDTA). The EDTA ensured that the sample did not clot, and that there was adequate plasma for analysis of hematocrit (needed for calculation of RBC folate later). The tube was then gently shaken to mix the blood and the anticoagulant. The serum folate sample was put in a tube without an anticoagulant to allow cells to separate from the serum after clotting. This tube had a gel to separate the red cells from the serum after the clotting of cells. The samples were kept at room temperature for 2–6 h, until they were transferred to a laboratory outside the Bwaila maternity wing (research site hospital) at the African Bible College Clinic—Center for Medical Diagnostics (CMED). At CMED, the RBC folate blood sample was centrifuged and frozen, kept at −80 °C until transfer by air to South Africa.

The folic acid analysis was done in South Africa by Lancet laboratories (Lancet, Johannesburg, South Africa) using ARCHITECT assay kits (Abbott Ireland, Longford, Ireland) on the ARCHITECT *i* system. The hemoglobin measurements were taken at bedside using a Hemocue Hb 201+ (HemoCue America, Brea, CA, USA).

2.6. Statistical Analyses

All data analyses were conducted using SPSS version 24 (SPSS Inc., Armonk, NY, USA) and SAS version 9.4 (SAS Institute, Cary, NC, USA). Descriptive statistics were used to calculate frequencies and mean and standard deviation values of variables. We also determined associations between maternal health and compliance to IFA factors, and hemoglobin and folate status using correlation analyses. Finally, multivariable logistic regression models were used to determine the degree of influence of iron and folic acid supplements on LBW infants as an outcome after controlling for covariates. Covariates were maternal age, education, total number of pregnancies, first prenatal visit trimester, and total number of prenatal visits.

3. Results

Table 1 shows that the mothers' age, residence, gravidity (number of pregnancies), parity, number of prenatal care clinic visits, and trimester of starting intake of IFA pills did not differ between mothers who gave birth to normal weight versus LBW newborns. Factors that differentiated the two groups were trimester of first prenatal clinic visit ($p = 0.003$) and gestation age ($p < 0.001$).

Table 1. Characteristics between mothers of normal weight and low birth weight newborns.

	Birth Weight of Newborn				
	Normal Weight (*n* = 179)		Low Birth Weight (*n* = 34)		
	N	%	N	%	*p* Value
Age					
<30 y	138	77.1	27	79.4	0.767
≥30 y	41	22.9	7	20.6	
Residence					
Rural	58	32.4	12	35.3	0.722
Peri-Urban	68	38.0	12	35.3	
Urban	53	29.6	10	29.4	
Gravidity					
1	54	30.3	16	47.1	0.058
≥2	124	69.7	18	52.9	
Missing	1				
Parity					
0	55	30.7	15	45.5	0.098
≥1	124	69.3	18	54.6	
Missing	1				
Gestation Weeks					
<37	38	24.1	22	71.0	<0.001
≥37	120	76.0	9	29.0	
Missing	24				
Education Level					
≤Primary	98	54.8	24	70.6	0.087
≥Secondary	81	45.3	10	29.4	
Trimester of First Prenatal Visit					
First	11	6.2	7	21.9	0.003
Second	134	75.3	23	71.9	
Third	33	18.5	2	6.3	
Missing	3				
No. of Prenatal Clinic Visits					
<4	97	55.8	21	63.6	0.401
≥4	77	44.3	12	36.4	
Missing	6				
No. of IFA Pills Taken during Pregnancy					
<45	17	54.8	64	36.6	0.084
45–89	12	38.7	77	44.0	
≥90	2	6.5	34	19.4	
Missing	7				
Trimester IFA Pill Intake Started					
First	13	8.4	7	25.0	0.088
Second	126	81.3	18	64.3	
Third	16	10.3	3	10.7	
Missing	30				

IFA, iron and folic acid; *p*-value by Chi-square test.

Table 2 shows a comparison of mothers' variables between normal weight and LBW newborns. Mean hemoglobin status between mothers of normal weight and LBW newborns were 11.4 ± 1.6 g/dL and 9.4 ± 1.6 g/dL ($p < 0.001$), respectively. The difference in serum folate between mothers of normal weight and LBW newborns was not significant—9.1 ± 4.4 nmol/L and 7.5 ± 3.6 nmol/L, respectively (*p* = 0.230). The same was observed with RBC folate status between normal weight and LBW—494.6 ± 413 nmol/L and 489.8 ± 181.1 nmol/L, respectively (*p* = 0.942).

Table 2. Differences in characteristics between mothers of normal weight and low birth weight newborns.

	Birth Weight						
	Normal Weight (*n* = 179)			Low Birth Weight (*n* = 34)			
	N	Mean	SD	N	Mean	SD	*p* Value
Mother's Variables							
Body Weight-1 (kg)	159	60.1	9.9	26	54.6	8.4	0.008
Body Weight-2 (kg)	125	66.4	11.2	16	59.5	8.6	0.019
Height (cm)	154	155.5	5.6	31	151.0	6.4	<0.001
Hb-1 (g/dL)	23	9.7	1.4	6	7.6	1.7	0.005
Hb-2 (g/dL)	172	11.4	1.6	27	9.4	1.6	<0.001
Serum Folate (nmol/L)	87	9.1	4.4	14	7.5	3.6	0.230
RBC Folate (nmol/L)	87	494.6	413.0	14	489.8	181.1	0.942
Placenta Weight (g)	145	591.4	129.2	26	455.6	153.9	<0.001

Body Weight-1: First prenatal visit weight, data were extracted from health passport book; Body Weight-2: Measured prior to delivery; Hb-1: Hemoglobin status at first prenatal clinic visit, data was extracted from health passport book; Hb-2: Hemoglobin level measured prior to delivery; IFA, iron and folic acid.

IFA pills taken by the women during pregnancy and the mean maternal hemoglobin levels before pregnancy are shown in Figure 1. Maternal hemoglobin levels were positively associated with the number of IFA pills taken. Mean hemoglobin levels were 10.7 g/dL, 11.3 g/dL, and 11.7 g/dL in response to the reported number of IFA pills taken from <45, 45–89, to ≥90, respectively (*p* = 0.006).

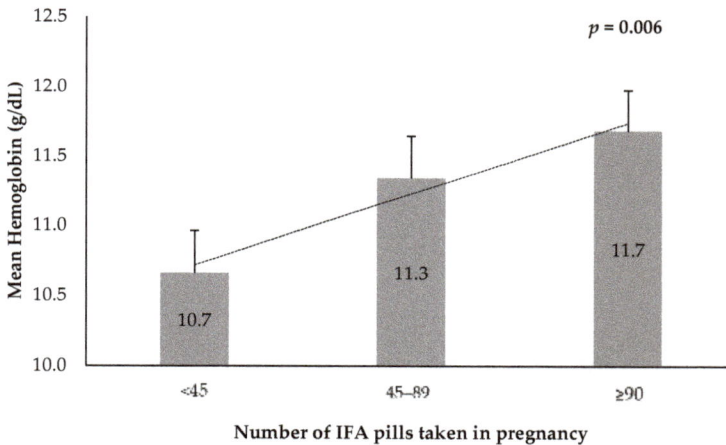

Figure 1. Mean maternal hemoglobin levels before delivery, by number of IFA pills taken during pregnancy.

The correlation of IFA pills taken with mothers' height, maternal hemoglobin, and serum folate were positive with a Spearman's correlation coefficient of 0.1759 (*p* = 0.019); 0.1846 (*p* = 0.010); and 0.1839 (*p* = 0.070), respectively (Table 3). The results of multivariable odds ratio (OR) for LBW and IFA pills intake and other variables are shown in Table 4. The OR was not significant for age categories, residence, gravidity, parity, education levels, number of prenatal clinic visits, and trimester of starting IFA pill intake. IFA supplement intake during pregnancy reduced the risk of delivering a LBW newborn. Women who took more than 60 IFA pills had lower risk (OR = 0.15, CI: 0.03, 0.70, *p* = 0.033) compared with the reference group who took ≤30 pills after controlling for maternal age, education, total number of pregnancies, first prenatal visit trimester, and total number of prenatal visits. Risk of LBW was lower for a gestation age $\geq$37 week (OR = 0.13, CI: 0.05, 0.35, p < 0.001) than a gestation age <37 weeks. Women who started prenatal care visit in the second or third trimester had a lower OR of LBW (OR = 0.16, CI: 0.05, 0.51, p = 0.002) compared to those who started in the first trimester.

Table 3. Spearman's correlation of prenatal iron and folic acid (IFA) supplement use with maternal characteristics.

		Body Weight-1	Body Weight-2	Height	Hemo-Globin	Serum Folate	RBC Folate
No. of IFA Pills	Corr. Coeff.	0.0599	0.0042	0.1759	0.1846	0.1839	−0.0329
	p value	0.426	0.961	0.019	0.010	0.070	0.748
	n	179	136	178	193	98	98
Body Weight-1	Corr. Coeff.		0.8910	0.1794	0.1025	0.0697	0.0266
	p value		<0.001	0.022	0.180	0.526	0.809
	n		129	164	173	85	85
Body Weight-2	Corr. Coeff.			0.2121	0.1489	0.0537	−0.0287
	p value			0.015	0.084	0.654	0.811
	n			131	136	72	72
Height	Corr. Coeff.				0.1819	−0.1529	−0.0432
	p value				0.016	0.141	0.679
	n				174	94	94
Hemoglobin	Corr. Coeff.					0.3905	−0.0167
	p value					<0.001	0.869
	n					100	100
Serum Folate	Corr. Coeff.						0.2502
	p value						0.012
	n						101

Body Weight-1: First prenatal visit weight, data were extracted from health passport book; Body Weight-2: Measured prior to delivery; Hemoglobin, serum and RBC folate samples were taken prior to delivery.

Table 4. Multivariable odds ratios (OR) and 95% confidence intervals (CIs) of low birth weight by its risk factors.

	Low Birth Weight			
	OR *	95% CI		p Value
Age (n = 204)				
<30 y	1.00			
$\geq$30 y	1.55	0.53	4.56	0.427
Residence (n = 204)				
Rural	1.00			
Peri-Urban	1.14	0.44	2.93	0.673
Urban	0.90	0.32	2.54	0.717
Gravidity (n = 204)				
1	1.00			
$\geq$2	0.45	0.18	1.14	0.093
Parity (n = 204)				
0	1.00			
$\geq$1	0.49	0.19	1.26	0.14
Gestation Weeks (n = 181)				
<37	1.00			
$\geq$37	0.13	0.05	0.35	<0.001
Education (n = 204)				
$\leq$Primary	1.00			
$\geq$Secondary	0.67	0.29	1.55	0.346
First ANC Visit Trimester (n = 204)				
First	1.00			
Second/Third	0.16	0.05	0.51	0.002

Table 4. *Cont.*

	Low Birth Weight		
	OR *	95% CI	*p* Value
No. of Prenatal Clinic Visits (*n* = 204)			
<4	1.00		
≥4	0.51	0.21 1.23	0.13
Trimester IFA Supplements Started (*n* = 159)			
First	1.00		
Second/Third	0.41	0.11 1.63	0.208
No. of IFA Pills Taken in Pregnancy (*n* = 199)			
≤30	1.00		
31–60	0.57	0.23 1.41	0.447
>60	0.15	0.03 0.70	0.033
No. of IFA Pills Taken in Pregnancy (*n* = 199)			
<45	1.00		
45–89	0.54	0.22 1.32	0.842
≥90	0.24	0.05 1.14	0.145

ANC, antenatal care; IFA, iron and folic acid. * Adjusted for maternal age, education, total number of pregnancies, first prenatal visit trimester, and total number of prenatal visits.

4. Discussion

The present study reported that the self-reported intake of IFA reduced the risk of LBW. Women who took more than 60 IFA supplements (pills) had significantly lower odds of delivering LBW babies, compared with pregnant women who took ≤30 pills. The more prenatal IFA pills were taken by pregnant women, the lower the risk of LBW. Similarly, a study by Nisar and colleagues, which used nationally representative data of Pakistan (demographic and health survey), found that self-reported intake of IFA pills of any amount during pregnancy was positively associated with better perceived birth size and birth weight. Any amount of IFA pills taken was associated with a reduced risk (by 18%) of having a smaller-than-average newborn [22]. Another study in India, which also used a national data set to examine the relationship between self-reported intake of IFA pills in pregnancy and LBW risk, found an inverse association. They found that at the population level, in a context where the burden of anemia is severe (prevalence ≥ 40%), IFA pills taken during pregnancy were significantly associated with low LBW. They concluded that the measures to improve the implementation of the prenatal supplementation program would likely help address India's burden of LBW [23]. The situation in India applies to Malawi because they are both developing countries with existing food security challenges in its communities, have a high prevalence of anemia, and prenatal IFA supplements have proven to be effective.

The compliance to prenatal IFA supplement use among pregnant women was directly associated with increased levels of maternal hemoglobin in the current study. This is in agreement with many other studies that show that maternal hemoglobin has modifying effects on infant birth weight in women receiving prenatal iron-containing supplements [8]. In a randomized double blind multicenter clinical trial (*n* = 18,775 participants) in China, it was found that supplementation of iron and folic acid, folic acid alone, or multiple micronutrient supplements (formulated by the United Nations) impacted birth weight, depending on hemoglobin status of the pregnant woman. Folic acid did not have much impact on birth weight; perhaps, this could explain our results above that although there is a positive association, it was not a statistically significant relationship. The supplement has to have a significant change on maternal hemoglobin levels, and hemoglobin modifies the birth weight of the newborn [8], with more impact seen in those with better hemoglobin status at baseline. Those receiving folic acid supplements alone did not have significant better birth outcomes but those with combined pills or multiple micronutrients did. Another study showed that supplementation did not just improve newborn anthropometric measurements, but also reduced the prevalence of anemia in mothers [12]. Steer also found that low hemoglobin is associated with LBW [10].

We found that pregnant women who self-reported taking supplements consistently (at least two months) lowered their risk of delivering a LBW newborn significantly. After establishing that IFA impacts biomarkers of the hematological status of pregnant women and that biomarkers of supplement use (hemoglobin and folate) have modifying effects on birth weight, we wanted to examine if birth outcomes could be linked to "self-reported" IFA use during pregnancy. If self-reported use of IFA pills during pregnancy is validated to predict birth outcomes in Malawi, it could strengthen the lessons given in prenatal clinics as a part of the anemia prevention program. It could also help reduce the cost of a routine hemoglobin check, which are rarely done due to the lack of resources in Malawi (only 30 out 213 women had their hemoglobin levels tested during prenatal care).

In the present study, pregnant women whose prenatal care began in the second or third trimester had a lower risk of delivering LBW infants, compared to those whose prenatal care began in the first trimester. Most pregnant women in Malawi visit prenatal care clinics in the second trimester. Those who visit in the first trimester are more likely to have medical problems and commence prenatal care immediately after treatment of those issues. Therefore, the cause for LBW in these babies is likely a medical problem, which necessitated early prenatal care. However, there were women without issues in early pregnancy who stayed home until the second trimester and delivered healthier babies because of a healthy pregnancy; this may not necessarily be due to the timing of the first prenatal care visit.

The biggest challenge identified was sustained intake of IFA pills longer than three months. Most pregnant women reported negligence, reduced supply of IFA supplements, and late start of prenatal clinic attendance as major reasons for poor compliance. Now that we have demonstrated that self-reported intake of prenatal supplements is a valid tool to predict hematological status of biomarkers and birth out comes of pregnant women, it is high time that a monitoring mechanism is put in place to evaluate pregnant women's compliance to IFA every time they visit a prenatal clinic. The monitoring mechanism could combine pill counting [18] to ensure that compliance is being achieved and pregnant women adhere to intake of IFA pills supplements. Pill counting has been employed successfully to improve adherence to ant-retroviral drugs in the treatment of HIV/AIDS [24]. Another method being used in Malawi is directly observed treatment (DOT), where a patient takes drugs under the observation of a medical practitioner or a trusted guardian. DOT is being used in the treatment of tuberculosis (the first two weeks) and malaria prophylaxis in pregnant women at the prenatal clinic. An effective monitoring and evaluation mechanism would make the people of Malawi realize the benefits of the IFA supplementation program and make it more successful in lowering the prevalence of LBW. The education of pregnant women on the benefits of IFA on their newborns would also yield positive results, because negligence was one of the major reasons for poor compliance. Lowering the risk of LBW has long-term benefits, such as reducing infant and child mortality, decreasing stunting prevalence, which in turn has economic returns and national development [25].

Maternal nutrition status is a major determinant of LBW; however, social and demographic factors have also been reported as significant [26,27]. Muula et al. found in 2008 that maternal education was associated with birth weight. Those with low levels of education are more likely to have a LBW children than those with a higher education [26]. It was also found that parity was a factor of LBW, i.e., the first delivery was likely to be LBW, compared to later born children. The Malawi Demographic and Health Survey demonstrates that birth orders as well as the maternal age are factors for LBW. The firstborn child is likely to have low weight than the second, and younger mothers and those giving birth after 35 years of age are more likely to deliver a LBW child [6]. The wealth index of the family had a positive association with birth weight, as well as attainment of secondary education and location of residence (for example, cities vs. rural areas) [27].

The significance of this study is that the validation of the self-reported intake of IFA with biomarkers (Hb and serum and red blood cell folate) evaluated the effectiveness of the program in general in improving the health of women and birth outcomes, and monitoring approaches used by the Malawi government for the largest anemia program in the country. This research provides feedback to government programs and non-profit organizations working in nutrition in Malawi on the efficacy of prenatal supplements to reduce LBW. Overall, the research results provide evidence that the self-reported intake of IFA by pregnant women can be used as a monitoring tool for compliance to prenatal supplements. The study also introduces the innovation of using the placenta, which is normally discarded in Malawi, to determine compliance to and efficacy of prenatal supplements taken during pregnancy and its impact on newborn health.

5. Conclusions

In conclusion, self-reported IFA supplement intake in pregnancy is a predictor of birth weight. Compliance to prenatal IFA supplement use can be improved if the Malawian government improves the supply of IFA pills in clinics, ensures that every pregnant woman attends prenatal clinics early in pregnancy, and possibly adds pill count to the questions asked at a follow up before supplying the next batch of IFA pills. Further studies using a more nationally representative sample of pregnant women should be done to determine compliance to IFA and birth outcomes in Malawi.

Author Contributions: Conceptualization: A.T.C. and W.O.S. Manuscript writing: A.T.C. and W.O.S. Data analysis: A.T.C, D.S., S.S. Manuscript—Reviewing/Editing: A.T.C., D.S., S.S.C., S.S. and W.O.S. All authors have approved the final version of the manuscript.

Funding: The research was funded by grants from the MasterCard Foundation Scholars Program and the Department of Food Science and Human Nutrition at Michigan State University.

Acknowledgments: Aaron Thokozani Chikakuda was a MasterCard Scholar at Michigan State University, which was supported by the Master Card Foundation.

Conflicts of Interest: The authors declare no conflict of interest.

Abbreviations

LBW	low birth weight
IFA	iron and folic acid
Hb	Hemoglobin
RBC	red blood cell
OR	odds ratios

References

1. Arnold, L.; Hoy, W.; Wang, Z. Low birthweight increases risk for cardiovascular disease hospitalisations in a remote Indigenous Australian community—A prospective cohort study. *Aust. N. Z. J. Public Health* **2016**, *40*, S102–S106. [CrossRef] [PubMed]
2. Smith, C.; Ryckman, K.; Barnabei, V.; Howard, B.; Isasi, C.R.; Sarto, G.; Tom, S.; Van Horn, L.; Wallace, R.; Robinson, J. The impact of birth weight on cardiovascular disease risk in the Women's Health Initiative. *Nutr. Metab. Cardiovasc. Dis.* **2016**, *26*, 239–245. [CrossRef] [PubMed]
3. McCormick, M.C. The contribution of low birth weight to infant mortality and childhood morbidity. *N. Engl. J. Med.* **1985**, *312*, 82–90. [CrossRef] [PubMed]
4. Wardlaw, T.M.; Blanc, A.; Zupan, J.; Ahman, A. *Low Birthweight: Country, Regional and Global Estimates*; UNICEF: New York, NY, USA, 2004.
5. Lau, C.; Ambalavanan, N.; Chakraborty, H.; Wingate, M.S.; Carlo, W.A. Extremely low birth weight and infant mortality rates in the United States. *Pediatrics* **2013**, *131*, 855–860. [CrossRef] [PubMed]
6. NSO-ICF. *Malawi Demographic and Health Survey 2015–2016*; National Statistical Office (NSO): Zomba, Malawi; ICF: Rockville, MD, USA, 2017. Available online: https://dhsprogram.com/pubs/pdf/FR319/FR319.pdf (accessed on 8 March 2017).
7. Abubaker, M.S. Anaemia and low birth weight in Medani, Hospital Sudan. *BMC Res. Notes* **2016**, *3*, 181. [CrossRef]

8.	Wang, L.; Mei, Z.; Li, H.; Zhang, Y.; Liu, J.; Serdula, M.K. Modifying effects of maternal Hb concentration on infant birth weight in women receiving prenatal iron-containing supplements: A randomised controlled trial. *Br. J. Nutr.* **2016**, *115*, 644–649. [CrossRef] [PubMed]

9.	Bhutta, Z.A.; Ahmed, T.; Black, R.E.; Cousens, S.; Dewey, K.; Giugliani, E.; Haider, B.A.; Kirkwood, B.; Morris, S.S.; Sachdev, H. What works? Interventions for maternal and child undernutrition and survival. *Lancet* **2008**, *371*, 417–440. [CrossRef]

10.	Steer, P.J. Maternal hemoglobin concentration and birth weight. *Am. J. Clin. Nutr.* **2000**, *71*, 1285S–1287S. [CrossRef] [PubMed]

11.	Haider, B.A.; Olofin, I.; Wang, M.; Spiegelman, D.; Ezzati, M.; Fawzi, W.W. Anaemia, prenatal iron use, and risk of adverse pregnancy outcomes: Systematic review and meta-analysis. *BMJ* **2013**, *346*, f3443. [CrossRef] [PubMed]

12.	Preziosi, P.; Prual, A.; Galan, P.; Daouda, H.; Boureima, H.; Hercberg, S. Effect of iron supplementation on the iron status of pregnant women: Consequences for newborns. *Am. J. Clin. Nutr.* **1997**, *66*, 1178–1182. [CrossRef] [PubMed]

13.	Owens, S.; Gulati, R.; Fulford, A.J.; Sosseh, F.; Denison, F.C.; Brabin, B.J.; Prentice, A.M. Periconceptional multiple-micronutrient supplementation and placental function in rural Gambian women: A double-blind, randomized, placebo-controlled trial. *Am. J. Clin. Nutr.* **2015**, *102*, 1450–1459. [CrossRef] [PubMed]

14.	Rwebembera, A.A.-B.; Munubhi, E.; Manji, K.; Mpembeni, R.; Philip, J. Relationship between infant birth weight ≤2000 g and maternal zinc levels at Muhimbili National Hospital, Dar Es Salaam, Tanzania. *J. Trop. Pediatr.* **2006**, *52*, 118–125. [CrossRef] [PubMed]

15.	Makrides, M.; Crowther, C.A.; Gibson, R.A.; Gibson, R.S.; Skeaff, C.M. Efficacy and tolerability of low-dose iron supplements during pregnancy: A randomized controlled trial. *Am. J. Clin. Nutr.* **2003**, *78*, 145–153. [CrossRef] [PubMed]

16.	Timmermans, S.; Jaddoe, V.W.; Hofman, A.; Steegers-Theunissen, R.P.; Steegers, E.A. Periconception folic acid supplementation, fetal growth and the risks of low birth weight and preterm birth: The Generation R Study. *Br. J. Nutr.* **2009**, *102*, 777–785. [CrossRef] [PubMed]

17.	Sharma, S.R.; Giri, S.; Timalsina, U.; Bhandari, S.S.; Basyal, B.; Wagle, K.; Shrestha, L. Low birth weight at term and its determinants in a tertiary hospital of Nepal: A case-control study. *PLoS ONE* **2015**, *10*, e0123962. [CrossRef] [PubMed]

18.	Young, M.; Lupafya, E.; Kapenda, E.; Bobrow, E. The effectiveness of weekly iron supplementation in pregnant women of rural northern Malawi. *Trop. Doct.* **2000**, *30*, 84–88. [CrossRef] [PubMed]

19.	Kalimbira, A.; Mtimuni, B.; Chilima, D. Maternal knowledge and practices related to anaemia and iron supplementation in rural Malawi: A cross-sectional study. *Afr. J. Food Agric. Nutr. Dev.* **2009**, *9*, 550–564. [CrossRef]

20.	Abioye, A.I.; Aboud, S.; Premji, Z.; Etheredge, A.J.; Gunaratna, N.S.; Sudfeld, C.R.; Mongi, R.; Meloney, L.; Darling, A.M.; Noor, R.A. Iron Supplementation Affects Hematologic Biomarker Concentrations and Pregnancy Outcomes among Iron-Deficient Tanzanian Women. *J. Nutr.* **2016**, *146*, 1162–1171. [CrossRef] [PubMed]

21.	Ahmed, E.B.; Ali, E.A.; Mohamed, E.H.; Saleh, E.A.; Elbaset, A.K.A.; Mahmmed, E.M.; Elaal, A.S.A.; Elsayed, A.M.; Quora, A.F.; Hashem, Z.M. Assessment of iron and calcium supplements compliance among pregnant women attending antenatal care unit of Al-Sabah Banat primary health care unit in Ismailia, Egypt. *J. Med. Biol. Sci. Res.* **2015**, *1*, 24–29.

22.	Nisar, Y.B.; Dibley, M.J. Antenatal iron–folic acid supplementation reduces risk of low birthweight in Pakistan: Secondary analysis of Demographic and Health Survey 2006–2007. *Matern. Child Nutr.* **2016**, *12*, 85–98. [CrossRef] [PubMed]

23.	Balarajan, Y.; Subramanian, S.; Fawzi, W.W. Maternal iron and folic acid supplementation is associated with lower risk of low birth weight in India. *J. Nutr.* **2013**, *143*, 1309–1315. [CrossRef] [PubMed]

24.	Dasgupta, A.N.; Wringe, A.; Crampin, A.C.; Chisambo, C.; Koole, O.; Makombe, S.; Sungani, C.; Todd, J.; Church, K. HIV policy and implementation: A national policy review and an implementation case study of a rural area of northern Malawi. *AIDS Care* **2016**, *28*, 1097–1109. [CrossRef] [PubMed]

25.	Win, A.Z. Micronutrient deficiencies in early childhood can lower a country's GDP: The Myanmar example. *Nutrition* **2016**, *32*, 138–140. [CrossRef] [PubMed]

26. Muula, A.; Siziya, S.; Rudatsikira, E. Parity and maternal education are associated with low birth weight in Malawi. *Afr. Health Sci.* **2011**, *11*, 65–71. [PubMed]

27. Ngwira, A.; Stanley, C.C. Determinants of low birth weight in Malawi: Bayesian geo-additive modelling. *PLoS ONE* **2015**, *10*, e0130057. [CrossRef] [PubMed]

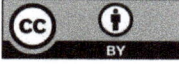

nutrients

MDPI

Article

Longitudinal Maternal Vitamin D Status during Pregnancy Is Associated with Neonatal Anthropometric Measures

Ellen C. Francis [1,2], Stefanie N. Hinkle [1], Yiqing Song [3], Shristi Rawal [1,4], Sarah R. Donnelly [1,5], Yeyi Zhu [6], Liwei Chen [2] and Cuilin Zhang [1,*]

[1] Epidemiology Branch, Division of Intramural Population Health Research, Eunice Kennedy Shriver National Institute of Child Health and Human Development, National Institutes of Health, Bethesda, MD 20892, USA; ellen.francis@NIH.gov (E.C.F.); stefanie.hinkle@nih.gov (S.N.H.); shristi.rawal@rutgers.edu (S.R.); srdonnelly04@vt.edu (S.R.D.)
[2] Department of Public Health Sciences, Clemson University, Clemson, SC 29634, USA; ecfranc@clemson.edu or liweic@clemson.edu
[3] Department of Epidemiology, Indiana University Richard M. Fairbanks School of Public Health, Indianapolis, IN 47405, USA; yiqsong@iu.edu
[4] Department of Nutritional Sciences, Rutgers School of Health Professions, Newark, NJ 07102, USA
[5] Department of Human Nutrition, Foods, and Exercise, Virginia Tech, Blacksburg VA 24061, USA
[6] Division of Research, Kaiser Permanente Northern California, Oakland, CA 94612 USA; yeyi.zhu@kp.org
*   Correspondence: zhangcu@mail.nih.gov; Tel.: +1-301-435-6917

check for updates

Received: 11 October 2018; Accepted: 26 October 2018; Published: 2 November 2018

Abstract: Findings on maternal 25-hydroxyvitamin D (25[OH]D) and neonatal anthropometry are inconsistent, and may at least be partly due to variations in gestational week (GW) of 25(OH)D measurement and the lack of longitudinal 25(OH)D measurements across gestation. The aim of the current study was to examine the associations of longitudinal measures of maternal 25(OH)D and neonatal anthropometry at birth. This study included 321 mother–offspring pairs enrolled in the *Eunice Kennedy Shriver* National Institute of Child Health and Human Development Fetal Growth Studies–Singletons. This study was a prospective cohort design without supplementation and without data on dietary supplementation. Nevertheless, measurement of plasma 25(OH)D reflects vitamin D from different sources, including supplementation. Maternal concentrations of total 25(OH)D were measured at 10–14, 15–26, 23–31, and 33–39 GW and categorized as <50 nmol/L, 50–75 nmol/L, and >75 nmol/L. Generalized linear models were used to examine associations of 25(OH)D at each time-point with neonate birthweight z-score, length, and sum of skinfolds at birth. At 10–14 GW, 16.8% and 49.2% of women had 25(OH)D <50 nmol/L and between 50–75 nmol/L, respectively. The association of maternal 25(OH)D with neonatal anthropometry differed by GW and women's prepregnancy BMI (normal (<25.0 kg/m^2), overweight/obese (25.0–44.9 kg/m^2)). All analyses were stratified by prepregnancy BMI status. Among women with an overweight/obese BMI, 25(OH)D <50 nmol/L at 10–14 GW was associated with lower birthweight z-score (0.56; 95% CI: −0.99, −0.13) and length (−1.56 cm; 95% CI: −3.07, −0.06), and at 23–31 GW was associated with shorter length (−2.77 cm; 95% CI: −13.38, −4.98) and lower sum of skinfolds (−9.18 mm; 95% CI: −13.38, −4.98). Among women with a normal BMI, 25(OH)D <50 nmol/L at 10–14 GW was associated with lower sum of skinfolds (−2.64 mm; 95% CI: −5.03, −0.24), at 23–31 GW was associated with larger birthweight z-scores (0.64; 95% CI: 0.03, 1.25), and at 33-39 GW with both higher birthweight z-score (1.22; 95% CI: 0.71, 1.73) and longer length (1.94 cm; 95% CI: 0.37, 3.52). Maternal 25(OH)D status during pregnancy was associated with neonatal anthropometric measures, and the associations were specific to GW of 25(OH)D measurement and prepregnancy BMI.

Keywords: vitamin D; neonate anthropometry; fetal growth; maternal; infant

1. Introduction

Although the classical function of vitamin D is to regulate calcium and phosphorus metabolism in the intestine and bone, recent findings indicate its important role in several other biochemical and physiological processes, including regulation of the immune system, cellular differentiation, and blood pressure [1]. In humans, 25(OH)D, the hydrolyzed form of vitamin D, is the predominant form of circulating vitamin D and is considered the clinical standard for measuring bioactive vitamin D status [2]. Maternal 25(OH)D levels during pregnancy have been considered critical for both maternal health and fetal development [2–6]. Lower maternal 25(OH)D levels have been associated with unfavorable fetal growth outcomes, such as low birth weight, shorter bone length, and small-for-gestational age (SGA) births in some, though not all studies [7–10]. The inconsistent results in the literature may be partially caused by differences in timing of 25(OH)D measurement; for example, some studies have measured maternal 25(OH)D concentration early in pregnancy at 11–13 gestational weeks (GW) [7], while others have been later in pregnancy at 28–32 GW [10].

Rapid cardiometabolic and hormonal changes during pregnancy results in dynamic alterations in maternal 25(OH)D metabolism and circulating concentrations throughout pregnancy [6]. There is some evidence from recent studies that 25(OH)D increases throughout pregnancy [11–14]. As such, the gestational age when maternal 25(OH)D is measured may play a role in different findings of the associations between 25(OH)D and neonatal anthropometry. To our knowledge, only one study has examined maternal 25(OH)D measured twice during pregnancy (before 16 GW and 24–28 GW) and only maternal 25(OH)D concentrations at 24–28 GW were inversely associated with newborn knee–heel length [9]. The lack of longitudinal data on maternal 25(OH)D status at multiple time-points throughout pregnancy has limited our understanding of the association between maternal vitamin D status, particularly at specific developmental windows, and fetal growth [15,16]. Therefore, the current study aimed to examine the longitudinal associations of maternal 25(OH)D concentrations at multiple time-points throughout pregnancy and neonatal anthropometry, including birthweight, length, and sum of skinfolds at birth.

2. Materials and Methods

2.1. Study Population

The current study was based on data from a nested case-control study within the *Eunice Kennedy Shriver* National Institute of Child Health and Human Development (NICHD) Fetal Growth Studies–Singletons (2009–2013) [17]. Between 8–13 GWs, low-risk pregnant women without a history of chronic or medical conditions (e.g., prepregnancy hypertension, autoimmune disorders) were enrolled and followed through delivery. Extensive details on study design and participant characteristics have been previously published [17]. Women were recruited from 12 clinics across the US: Columbia University (NY), New York Hospital, Queens (NY), Christiana Care Health System (DE), Saint Peter's University Hospital (NJ), Medical University of South Carolina (SC), University of Alabama (AL), Northwestern University (IL), Long Beach Memorial Medical Center (CA), University of California, Irvine (CA), Fountain Valley Hospital (CA), Women and Infants Hospital of Rhode Island (RI), and Tufts University (MA). Written consent was obtained from all participants and institutional Review Board approval was obtained for all participating clinical sites, the data coordinating center, and NICHD (09-CH-N152). This study was carried out following the rules of the Declaration of Helsinki. The current study included 321 mother–offspring pairs who had maternal vitamin D biomarkers measured throughout pregnancy. This nested case-control study comprised women with gestational diabetes mellitus (GDM) ($n = 107$) and controls ($n = 214$) matched at a ratio of 1:2 on maternal age (± 2 years), race/ethnicity, and GW (± 2 weeks) at blood collection.

2.2. Assessment of Maternal Vitamin D

As a planned component of the NICHD Fetal Growth Studies-Singletons, maternal biospecimens were collected four times during pregnancy (10–14, 15–26, 23–31, and 33–39 GW) [17]. Maternal plasma vitamin D biomarkers were measured for all GDM cases and controls at 10–14 and 15–26 GW. At 23–31 and 33–39 GWs, one of the two controls was randomly selected and biomarkers were assayed in this same control at the later time-points. Within the larger prospective cohort study, and within the nested case-control, no vitamin D supplementation was provided for study purposes. Plasma concentrations of 25(OH)D2 and 25(OH)D3 (ng/mL) were measured using liquid chromatography–mass spectrometry (LC–MS). Total 25(OH)D was calculated as the sum of 25(OH)D2 and 25(OH)D3 and reported in nmol/L using the conversion unit of 2.5 [18].

2.3. Assessment of Neonatal Anthropometric Measurements

Gestational age- and sex-specific birthweight z-scores were derived using birthweight abstracted from medical records [19]. Neonatal anthropometric measures were collected after delivery (median 1 day; interquartile range 1–2 days). Measurements were obtained in at least duplicate using standard protocol [20–22]. Neonatal crown–heel length (cm) was measured using an infantometer, and skinfold thickness (mm) was measured using a Lange skinfold caliper. Abdominal flank, anterior thigh, subscapular, and tricep skinfolds were summed (sum of skinfolds) as a measure of neonatal adiposity. One of the clinical sites used the incorrect calipers and, thus, participants from this site were excluded from skinfold analyses ($n = 12$).

2.4. Covariates

Maternal sociodemographic characteristics were collected from detailed questionnaires at enrollment. At enrollment (8–13 GW), prepregnancy body mass index kg/m^2 (BMI) was calculated based on self-reported weight and measured height. Self-reported weight was highly correlated with weight subsequently measured by study personnel during the enrollment visit (correlation coefficients of 0.97) [23]. Prepregnancy BMI was categorized as normal weight (<25.0), overweight (25.0–29.9), or obese (≥30.0). Physical activity (PA) was assessed at enrollment regarding habitual PA, and at subsequent study visits regarding PA since the prior visit [24]. Clinical centers were grouped into three categories based on latitude (southern ≤37° N; middle 38° N–40° N; northern >40° N latitude) [25]. Season of blood collection was categorized as winter (January–March), spring (April–June), summer (July–September), and fall (October–December).

2.5. Statistical Analysis

Sampling weights were applied to all analyses to represent the full NICHD Fetal Growth Studies–Singletons population and account for the oversampling of women with GDM in the case-control study [26,27]. Following visual inspection of the data and residuals, normality of distribution was confirmed and therefore parametric models were fitted to the data. Descriptive statistics were presented as weighted mean ± standard error (SE) for continuous variables, and frequency and weighted percent for categorical variables. Significant differences among descriptive statistics were based on *t*-test for continuous variables and chi-square for categorical variables, with both standard errors and *P*-values for differences based on robust variance estimates. Generalized linear models with robust SE were used to examine associations between maternal total 25(OH)D at each visit and neonatal anthropometric measures of birthweight z-score, length, and sum of skinfolds. A test for a linear trend across quartiles was performed by fitting the median value for each quartile as a continuous variable in generalized linear models. Additionally, restricted cubic splines were used to test for nonlinear associations between maternal 25(OH)D and neonatal anthropometry, but a nonlinear relationship was not found.

Maternal 25(OH)D was examined both continuously and categorically. Categories of 25(OH)D were examined based on the distribution at each visit (quartiles), and based on cutoffs of <50 nmol/L, 50–75 nmol/L, and >75 nmol/L [1]. Currently, there is no consensus for 25(OH)D deficiency specific to pregnancy; thus, commonly used cutoffs when assessing 25(OH)D in pregnant women were used [8,28] and that would result in an adequate sample size in each category based on the distribution of 25(OH)D in our sample. Neonatal anthropometric outcomes were treated as continuous variables.

All models were adjusted for maternal matching factors, including maternal age (continuous), race/ethnicity (non-Hispanic White, non-Hispanic Black, Hispanic, Asian and Pacific Islander), and GW at blood draw. Additional covariates included education (high-school degree or less, Associate degree, Bachelor degree), prepregnancy BMI (continuous), marital status (married/living with a partner or not), and insurance (private/managed care or Medicaid/other). Models of neonatal length and sum of skinfolds were further adjusted for the number of days between delivery and measurement date.

Several sensitivity analyses were conducted to test the robustness of findings. Analyses were stratified by offspring gender, prepregnancy BMI (normal versus overweight/obese), race/ethnicity (non-Hispanic Black versus not), and PA at enrollment (<median versus ≥ median level). To examine the change in 25(OH)D status across pregnancy, three profiles of 25(OH)D concentrations throughout pregnancy were determined: (1) Consistently <50 nmol/L, (2) an alternating status ranging across all concentration categories, and (3) consistently >75 nmol/L. In addition, controlling for gestational weight gain by taking the difference between the weight at each time-point and the woman's prepregnancy weight was explored. All analyses were implemented using SAS Version 9.4 (SAS Institute, Cary, NC, USA), with $\alpha < 0.05$ as the level of significance.

3. Results

The mean ± SE levels of maternal 25(OH)D were 68.9 (1.5) nmol/L at 10–14 GW, 76.2 (1.8) nmol/L at 15–26 GW, 80.9 (2.7) nmol/L at 23–31 GW, and 82.5 (3.1) nmol/L at 33–39 GW. The percentage of women with 25(OH)D <50 nmol/L changed throughout pregnancy, with 16.8% at 10–14 GW, 11.1% at 15–26 GW, 11.2% at 23–31 GW, and 8.3% at 33–39 GW. The mean ± SE birthweight z-score was 0.22 (0.07), neonatal length was 50.3 (0.23) cm, and sum of skinfolds was 19.7 (0.4) mm. At enrollment (10–14 GW), maternal 25(OH)D was associated with race/ethnicity, prepregnancy BMI, education, insurance type, marital status, and PA, but not with maternal age, parity, smoking, season, or clinic location (Table 1).

Table 1. Characteristics and maternal 25(OH)D nmol/L concentrations at enrollment [1].

Characteristics	N (%)	Total 25(OH) DMean ± SE	p
All	321	68.9 (1.5)	-
Age (mean age, years) [2]	28.2 ± 0.5	-	-
<25	54 (30.0)	65.1 ± 3.0	
25–29	85 (29.7)	70.6 ± 4.3	
30–34	97 (25.8)	67.4 ± 4.0	
≥35	85 (14.5)	76.1 ± 4.6	0.11
Race/ethnicity			
Non-Hispanic white	75 (30.9)	81.3 ± 2.7	
Non-Hispanic black	45 (23.3)	58.3 ± 4.2	
Hispanic	123 (27.2)	66.8 ± 3.4	
Asian/Pacific Islander	78 (18.5)	64.6 ± 4.1	<0.001

Table 1. *Cont.*

Characteristics	N (%)	Total 25(OH) DMean ± SE	p
Prepregnancy BMI (mean, kg/m²) [2]	25.8 ± 0.4	-	-
Normal	162 (56.1)	72.3 ± 2.1	
Overweight	91 (28.7)	61.6 ± 3.3	
Obese	68 (15.1)	66.1 ± 3.6	0.01
Education (degree)			
High school or less	81 (25.1)	66.0 ± 2.4	
Associates	117 (35.2)	64.6 ± 3.5	
Bachelor's or higher	123 (39.8)	74.6 ± 3.6	0.02
Insurance			
Private or managed care	211 (64.6)	71.1 ± 3.0	
Medicaid, other	108 (35.4)	64.9 ± 2.2	0.04
Marital Status			
Not married	62 (27.1)	62.9 ± 3.0	
Married/living with a partner	259 (72.9)	71.2 ± 3.5	0.02
Nulliparous			
Yes	144 (51.1)	69.3 ± 3.1	
No	177 (48.9)	68.4 ± 2.2	0.77
Physical activity MET score Type-Sports/exercise [2]	11.1 ± 0.78	-	-
≥50th percentile	165 (50.3)	73.8 ± 3.0	
<50th percentile	156 (49.7)	64.0 ± 2.1	0.002
Smoking 6 months prepregnancy			
Yes	5 (0.7)	73.4 ± 4.3	
No	316 (99.3)	68.9 ± 4.6	0.54 [3]
Season of study enrollment			
Winter	89 (33.3)	67.8 ± 2.7	
Fall	71 (20.1)	67.4 ± 4.2	
Spring	78 (21.2)	69.3 ± 4.2	
Summer	82 (25.4)	72.1 ± 4.2	0.72
Clinic Location			
Southern (≤37° N)	117 (37.7)	67.2 ± 2.6	
Middle (38° N–40° N)	145 (44.4)	67.7 ± 4.4	
Northern (>40° N)	59 (17.9)	70.8 ± 3.4	0.54

[1] Participant characteristics are presented as frequency (weighted percent), total 25(OH)D (nmol/L) are presented as mean ± SE. [2] Represents mean ± SE for a continuous variable. [3] *p*-value not based on robust variance estimates due to small cell size.

Associations of maternal 25(OH)D and neonatal anthropometry varied by maternal prepregnancy BMI status (Tables 2 and 3). There were no substantial differences from our main results when controlling for gestational weight gain, when examining profiles of 25(OH)D throughout gestation (Figure S1), or in stratified analyses by offspring gender, maternal race/ethnicity, PA level at enrollment, or GDM status. In the following sections, the results of maternal 25(OH)D levels categorized as <50 nmol/L, 50–70 nmol/L, and >75 nmol/L and stratified by maternal prepregnancy BMI status are presented. Results of maternal 25(OH)D levels categorized by quartiles in relation to neonatal anthropometry can be found in Table S1, unstratified results of 25(OH)D levels categorized as <50 nmol/L, 50–70 nmol/L, and >75 nmol/L can be found in Table S2, and frequencies of women with GDM in each 25(OH)D category can be found in Table S3.

3.1. Total 25(OH)D and Neonatal Birthweight Z-Score, Length, and Sum of Skinfold in Women with Prepregnancy Overweight/Obese BMI (>25 kg/m²)

Among women with prepregnancy overweight/obesity, maternal 25(OH)D was negatively associated with offspring birthweight z-score, length, and sum of skinfolds, but the strength of the association varied by exposure window during pregnancy (Table 2). At 10–14 GW, neonates of women with 25(OH)D <50 nmol/L had a lower birthweight ($p = 0.01$) and shorter length ($p = 0.04$) than neonates of women with 25(OH)D >75 nmol/L. At 23–31 GW, neonates of women with 25(OH)D <50 nmol/L had shorter length ($p = 0.001$) and lower sum of skinfolds ($p < 0.0001$) than neonates of women with 25(OH)D >75 nmol/L. At 33–39 GW, neonates of women with 25(OH)D <50 nmol/L had shorter length ($p = 0.02$) than neonates of women with 25(OH)D >75 nmol/L.

Table 2. Longitudinal associations of maternal total 25(OH)D (nmol/L) and birthweight z-score, length (cm), and sum of skinfolds (mm) among women with an overweight/obese prepregnancy BMI [1].

Maternal 25(OH)D Status	*n*	10–14 GW	*n*	15–26 GW	*n*	23–31 GW	*n*	33–39 GW
Birthweight z-score								
<50 nmol/L	45	−0.56 (−0.99, −0.13) *	24	0.15 (−0.51, 0.80)	11	−0.52 (−1.00, −0.04) *	12	−0.17 (−0.74, 0.40)
50–75 nmol/L	73	−0.35 (−0.68, −0.03) *	73	0.04 (−0.33, 0.41)	46	−0.13 (−0.58, 0.32)	43	0.29 (−0.17, 0.76)
>75 nmol/L	32	Reference	51	Reference	52	Reference	46	Reference
Length								
<50 nmol/L	27	−1.56 (−3.07, −0.06) *	22	0.98 (−1.01, 2.98)	11	−2.77 (−4.43, −1.12) *	11	−1.98 (−3.66, −0.31) *
50–75 nmol/L	6 8	−2.04 (−3.37, −0.71) *	64	1.06 (−0.61, 2.74)	43	−2.40 (−3.71, −1.08) *	38	1.76 (0.32, 3.19) *
>75 nmol/L	41	Reference	49	Reference	49	Reference	44	Reference
Sum of Skinfolds								
<50 nmol/L	25	−0.52 (−4.34, 3.30)	18	3.57 (−0.43, 7.57)	9	−9.18 (−13.38, −4.98) *	9	−4.29 (−8.75, 0.17)
50–75 nmol/L	63	0.69 (−2.30, 3.69)	63	4.94 (2.36, 7.52) *	43	−0.85 (−3.86, 2.17)	39	2.52 (−1.42, 6.46)
>75 nmol/L	37	Reference	44	Reference	46	Reference	40	Reference

[1] Data are presented as regression coefficients and confidence intervals (CI) and reflect the differences in neonatal anthropometry compared to the reference group (25(OH)D >75 nom/L). All models are adjusted for maternal matching characteristics (age (continuous), race, and gestational age at blood collection), and adjusted for education, insurance type, marital status, and prepregnancy BMI (continuous). Models of sum of skinfolds were adjusted to account for the difference in days between birth and date of anthropometric measurement. * (*p*-value < 0.005).

3.2. Total 25(OH)D and Neonatal Birthweight Z-Score, Length, and Sum of Skinfold in Women with Prepregnancy Normal BMI (18.5–24.9 kg/m²)

Among women with a normal prepregnancy BMI, the direction of associations of maternal 25(OH)D with neonatal anthropometry varied by exposure window during pregnancy (Table 3). At 10–14 GW, neonates of women who had 25(OH)D <50 nmol/L had lower sum of skinfolds ($p = 0.03$) than neonates of women with 25(OH)D >75 nmol/L; similar findings were observed for 25(OH)D concentrations between 50–75 nmol/L. At 23–31 GW, neonates of women with 25(OH)D <50 nmol/L had larger birthweight z-scores ($p = 0.04$) than neonates of women with 25(OH)D >75 nmol/L. At 33–39 GW, neonates of women with 25(OH)D <50 nmol/L had larger birthweight z-scores ($p < 0.0001$) and ($p = 0.02$) larger length compared to neonates of women with 25(OH)D >75 nmol/L.

Table 3. Longitudinal associations of maternal total 25(OH)D (nmol/L) and birthweight z-score, length (cm), and sum of skinfolds (mm) among women with a normal prepregnancy BMI [1].

Maternal 25(OH)D Status	n	10–14 GW	n	15–26 GW	n	23–31 GW	n	33–39 GW
Birthweight z-score								
<50 nmol/L	24	0.05 (−0.40, 0.51)	12	0.09 (−0.49, 0.67)	6	0.64 0.03, 1.25) *	3	1.22 (0.71, 1.73) *
50–75 nmol/L	65	−0.15 (−0.50, 0.20)	48	−0.26 (−0.59, 0.07)	22	0.08 (−0.49, 0.65)	26	−0.01 (−0.37, 0.34)
>75 nmol/L	67	Reference	94	Reference	64	Reference	57	Reference
Length								
<50 nmol/L	23	0.67 (−0.93, 2.28)	12	0.54 (−1.54, 2.62)	6	1.61 (−0.34, 3.55)	3	1.94 (0.37, 3.52) *
50–75 nmol/L	59	−0.24 (−1.32, 0.85)	44	−0.34 (−1.19, 0.52)	22	−0.47 (−1.59, 0.64)	26	0.19 (−0.89, 1.28)
>75 nmol/L	62	Reference	87	Reference	59	Reference	52	Reference
Sum of Skinfolds								
<50 nmol/L	19	−2.64 (−5.03, −0.24) *	11	−0.15 (−2.34, 2.05)	6	0.84 (−2.52, 4.21)	3	1.29 (−2.22, 4.80)
50–75 nmol/L	59	−2.32 (−4.00, −0.63) *	42	−1.42 (−3.04, 0.19)	20	−0.66 (−3.12, 1.80)	24	1.83 (−0.37, 4.03)
>75 nmol/L	60	Reference	84	Reference	58	Reference	53	Reference

[1] Data are presented as regression coefficients and confidence intervals (CI) and reflect the differences in neonatal anthropometry compared to the reference group (25(OH)D >75 nom/L). All models are adjusted for maternal matching characteristics (age (continuous), race, and gestational age at blood collection), and adjusted for education, insurance type, marital status, and prepregnancy BMI (continuous). Models of sum of skinfolds were adjusted to account for the difference in days between birth and date of anthropometric measurement. * (p-value < 0.005).

4. Discussion

In the current study, the direction of association between maternal 25(OH)D and neonatal anthropometry varied by maternal prepregnancy adiposity status and GW of 25(OH)D measurement. Although maternal 25(OH)D is recognized to play an important role in fetal growth, due to a lack of studies with longitudinal measures of 25(OH)D during pregnancy in relation to neonatal anthropometry, direct comparison of our results with previous findings is challenging. In the following sections, the congruency of our results based on the time-point during pregnancy when 25(OH)D was measured and neonatal outcome is discussed.

4.1. Maternal 25(OH)D and Neonatal Birthweight

Most studies reporting a positive association between maternal 25(OH)D and neonatal birthweight mostly included women with prepregnancy normal weight, limiting the comparability to our study [29,30]. A study that measured maternal 25(OH)D multiple times during pregnancy (11–16 and 28–32 GW) found no associations between 25(OH)D <28 nmol/L at either time-point and neonatal birthweight [9]. Although they controlled for maternal BMI, the mean BMI was not reported. Several other studies were based on a single time-point and used much lower cutoffs for 25(OH)D (i.e., <25 nmol/L), and reported a positive association between maternal 25(OH)D in later pregnancy and birthweight [31,32]. We are not aware of any observational studies that observed a negative association between maternal 25(OH)D after 32 GW and birthweight and thus our findings among women with normal weight require replication.

4.2. Maternal 25(OH)D and Neonatal Length

A previous study, which examined maternal 25(OH)D twice during pregnancy, found no association of 25(OH)D at 11–16 GW, but, similar to our results, found a positive association at 28–32 GW with neonatal length [9]. That study did not stratify by BMI or report the mean BMI and, thus, direct comparisons with our study are challenging. To our knowledge, no study has examined associations of maternal 25(OH)D in late pregnancy (>32 GW) and neonatal length. The finding of significant associations in late pregnancy (33–39 GW), regardless of prepregnancy BMI status, has not been previously reported and warrants confirmation.

4.3. Maternal 25(OH)D and Neonatal Sum of Skinfolds

Previously, a positive association between 25(OH)D measured at 28–32 GW and neonatal subscapular skinfold thickness was observed [9], but again, the adiposity status of the women was not reported. Contrary to our findings, a study among mostly women with normal weight found no association between maternal 25(OH)D at <26 GW and neonatal adiposity as measured by ponderal index [30].

Differences among study findings may be related to study design, population, timing when the maternal 25(OH)D was measured, and distribution of 25(OH)D concentrations. In some studies, there was a high proportion of women with extremely low concentrations of 25(OH)D [29,31–33], whereas in our study, less than 20% of women had 25(OH)D <50 nmol/L at any time during pregnancy. The increase in 25(OH)D throughout gestation is typical of the pregnant state and is in response to the physiological demands of pregnancy [2].

The exposure window during pregnancy when maternal 25(OH)D may impact neonatal size is important to consider in relation to fetal growth in utero. In early pregnancy, bones and muscles begin to grow, including the formation of arms, legs, backbone, and neck [34]. In late pregnancy, the fetus gains weight mainly through accumulation of fat mass and bone density [34]. Although the association of 25(OH)D and neonate anthropometry at birth was dependent on GW, there are many factors that contribute to fetal growth. It is likely the interplay of vitamin D with many other hormones and nutrients that results in the overall body composition of the neonate at birth. For instance, maternal calcium absorption and placental calcium transfer both increase to meet fetal demands and are responsive to 1,25(OH)$_2$D, the biologically active form of vitamin D [35]. Calcium serves as a key structural component in bone development, with higher concentrations needed for the fetus to effectively mineralize the skeleton [36]. The role of vitamin D in calcium absorption may therefore also impact fetal skeletal muscle and bone development. The concentration of calcium available to the fetus is heavily dependent on maternal concentrations, the latter of which has been reported to explain 3% of the variance in birth length [37]. Therefore, maternal vitamin D status, as reflected by 25(OH)D concentrations, may represent its role in skeletal function in fetal growth. On the other hand, adequate maternal vitamin D status has been favorably associated with improving maternal glucose and insulin homeostasis [38], which may have a downstream impact on the glucose load experienced by the fetus, which in turn may curb excessive fetal growth in late gestation. In addition, vitamin D's role in immune function, systemic inflammation, and endothelial function is important for normal placental function. Maternal concentrations of 25(OH)D may also stimulate secretion of placental hormones that facilitate fetal growth, such as placental lactogen [6].

Inverse associations of maternal 25(OH)D with birthweight and length among women with prepregnancy normal weight has not been reported before. In our study, women with prepregnancy overweight/obesity had lower 25(OH)D concentrations at enrollment than women with normal weight. The differences in synthesis and metabolism of vitamin D among individuals with and without obesity is still under investigation [39,40], and the impact of these differences on fetal growth is unclear.

4.4. Strengths and Limitations

The current study has several strengths, including prospective longitudinal data collection, thereby allowing the investigation of gestation-specific associations of maternal 25(OH)D and neonatal anthropometry. Data on plasma concentrations of 25(OH)D were used, which is downstream of supplement and dietary sources and has been reported to be the most accurate indicator of total exposure to vitamin D from all sources [3]. Moreover, study participants were enrolled from geographically diverse US clinics and represented various race/ethnicities. Detailed data on potential confounders during and prior to pregnancy were available and controlled for when appropriate, and interactions with offspring gender, race/ethnicity, and maternal prepregnancy BMI status were explored. Although we have controlled for known major confounders, similar to other observational studies, we cannot completely exclude the possibility for residual confounding by unmeasured factors or measurement errors. In the current study, there was a relatively small sample size, which precluded us from examining extreme phenotypes of fetal growth, such as small- or large-for-gestational age. Lastly, self-reported prepregnancy weight was used to calculate prepregnancy BMI upon recruitment into the cohort. However, self-reported weight was highly correlated with measured maternal weight (r = 0.97) in this population and other studies [23,41].

4.5. Suggestions for Future Research

In addition to investigating maternal 25(OH)D status during different time windows of pregnancy in association with neonatal anthropometry, our study further evaluated whether the impact of maternal vitamin D status on offspring anthropometric measures varied by maternal prepregnancy BMI (i.e., normal weight vs. overweight/obese), which has not been previously investigated in the literature. In the current study, there was a difference in direction of association between 25(OH)D and neonatal anthropometry by BMI categories (i.e., at 33–39 GW, there was an inverse association with length among women with a prepregnancy BMI in the normal range, but a positive association among women with a prepregnancy BMI in the overweight/obese range). Future investigations are warranted to replicate these findings. If confirmed, these findings indicate that endeavors to optimize maternal 25(OH)D status should likely consider women's prepregnancy adiposity status and the specific neonatal anthropometric outcome, both of which are justifications for efforts into precision nutrition.

5. Conclusions

If confirmed, our findings highlight the significance of the concept of precision nutrition, which considers tailored approaches to 25(OH)D supplementation to improve fetal outcomes by considering timing of GW and maternal adiposity status. At least among women who were overweight/obese before pregnancy, low 25(OH)D (<50 nmol/L) in both early and late pregnancy may impact fetal development. Considering that almost half of US women entering pregnancy are overweight or obese, prevention of low 25(OH)D concentrations in early and late pregnancy may be particularly relevant to optimizing fetal growth.

Supplementary Materials: The following are available online at http://www.mdpi.com/2072-6643/10/11/1631/s1, Table S1: Longitudinal associations of maternal total 25(OH)D and neonatal birthweight z-score, length (cm), and sum of skinfolds stratified by prepregnancy BMI1, Table S2: Longitudinal associations of maternal total 25(OH)D (nmol/L) and birthweight z-score, length (cm), and sum of skinfolds (mm), Table S3: Frequency of cases and controls by 25(OH)D status in the full sample and stratified by prepregnancy BMI, Figure S1: Association between 25(OH)D profiles and neonatal anthropometry.

Author Contributions: E.C.F. analyzed the data and wrote the first draft of the manuscript. S.N.H. contributed to the analysis and interpretation of the data and revised the manuscript. Y.S., S.R., S.R.D., Y.Z., and L.C. contributed to the interpretation and reviewed the manuscript. C.Z. obtained funding, designed and oversaw the study, and revised the manuscript. All authors interpreted the results, revised the manuscript for important intellectual content, and approved the final version of the manuscript. E.C.F. and C.Z. are the guarantors of this work and, as such, had full access to all the data in the study and take responsibility for the integrity of the data and the accuracy of the data analysis.

Funding: This research was supported by the *Eunice Kennedy Shriver* National Institute of Child Health and Human Development intramural funding and included American Recovery and Reinvestment Act funding via contract numbers HHSN275200800013C, HHSN275200800002I, HHSN27500006, HHSN275200800003IC, HHSN275200800014C, HHSN275200800012C, HHSN275200800028C, HHSN275201000009C, and HHSN275201000001Z. Zhu was supported by a mentored research scientist development award from the National Institutes of Health Office of the Director and the Building Interdisciplinary Research Careers in Women's Health program (3K12HD052163).

Acknowledgments: Ellen C. Francis is a participant in the National Institute of Health Graduate Partnership Program and a graduate student at Clemson University

Conflicts of Interest: The authors declare no conflict of interest.

Abbreviations

BMI	Body Mass Index
CI	Confidence Interval
GDM	Gestational Diabetes Mellitus
GW	Gestational Week
PA	Physical Activity
SE	Standard Error
25[OH]D	Total 25-hydroxyvitamin D calculated as $25[OH]D_2$ + $25[OH]D_3$
$25[OH]D_3$	25-hydroxycholecalciferol
$25[OH]D_2$	25-hydroxyergocalciferol

References

1. Holick, M.F. Vitamin D deficiency. *N. Eng. J. Med.* **2007**, *357*, 266–281. [CrossRef] [PubMed]
2. Wagner, C.L.; Taylor, S.N.; Dawodu, A.; Johnson, D.D.; Hollis, B.W. Vitamin D and Its Role During Pregnancy in Attaining Optimal Health of Mother and Fetus. *Nutrients* **2012**, *4*, 208–230. [CrossRef] [PubMed]
3. Brannon, P.M.; Picciano, M.F. Vitamin D in pregnancy and lactation in humans. *Annu. Rev. Nutr.* **2011**, *31*, 89–115. [CrossRef] [PubMed]
4. Hollis, B.W.; Wagner, C.L. Vitamin D supplementation during pregnancy: Improvements in birth outcomes and complications through direct genomic alteration. *Mol. Cell. Endocrinol.* **2017**, *453*, 113–130. [CrossRef] [PubMed]
5. Abrams, S.A. Vitamin D supplementation during pregnancy. *J. Bone Miner. Res.* **2011**, *26*, 2338–2340. [CrossRef] [PubMed]
6. Shin, J.S.; Choi, M.Y.; Longtine, M.S.; Nelson, D.M. Vitamin D effects on pregnancy and the placenta. *Placenta* **2010**, *31*, 1027–1034. [CrossRef] [PubMed]
7. Ertl, R.; Yu, C.K.H.; Samaha, R.; Akolekar, R.; Nicolaides, K.H. Maternal Serum Vitamin D at 11-13 Weeks in Pregnancies Delivering Small for Gestational Age Neonates. *Fetal Diagnosis Ther.* **2012**, *31*, 103–108. [CrossRef] [PubMed]
8. Aghajafari, F.; Nagulesapillai, T.; Ronksley, P.E.; Tough, S.C.; O'Beirne, M.; Rabi, D.M. Association between maternal serum 25-hydroxyvitamin D level and pregnancy and neonatal outcomes: Systematic review and meta-analysis of observational studies. *BMJ Br. Med. J.* **2013**, *346*, f1169. [CrossRef] [PubMed]
9. Morley, R.; Carlin, J.B.; Pasco, J.A.; Wark, J.D. Maternal 25-Hydroxyvitamin D and Parathyroid Hormone Concentrations and Offspring Birth Size. *J. Clin. Endocrinol. Metab.* **2006**, *91*, 906–912. [CrossRef] [PubMed]
10. Ong, Y.L.; Quah, P.L.; Tint, M.T.; Aris, J.M.; Chen, L.W.; Van Dam, R.M.; Heppe, D.; Saw, S.-M.; Godfrey, K.M.; Gluckman, P.D.; et al. The association of maternal vitamin D status with infant birth outcomes, postnatal growth and adiposity in the first 2 years of life in a multi-ethnic Asian population: The Growing Up in Singapore Towards healthy Outcomes (GUSTO) cohort study. *Br. J. Nutr.* **2016**, *116*, 621–631. [CrossRef] [PubMed]
11. Agudelo-Zapata, Y.; Maldonado-Acosta, L.M. Serum 25-hydroxyvitamin D levels throughout pregnancy: A longitudinal study in healthy and preeclamptic pregnant women. *Endocr. Connect* **2018**, *7*, 698–707. [CrossRef] [PubMed]
12. Lundqvist, A.; Sandström, H.; Stenlund, H.; Johansson, I.; Hultdin, J. Vitamin D Status during Pregnancy: A Longitudinal Study in Swedish Women from Early Pregnancy to Seven Months Postpartum. *PLoS ONE* **2016**, *11*, e0150385. [CrossRef] [PubMed]
13. Choi, R.; Kim, S.; Yoo, H.; Cho, Y.; Kim, S.; Chung, J.; Oh, S.; Lee, S. High prevalence of vitamin D deficiency in pregnant Korean women: The first trimester and the winter season as risk factors for vitamin D deficiency. *Nutrients* **2015**, *7*, 3427–3448. [CrossRef] [PubMed]
14. Milman, N.; Hvas, A.M.; Bergholt, T. Vitamin D status during normal pregnancy and postpartum. A longitudinal study in 141 Danish women. *J. Perinat. Med.* **2011**, *40*, 57–61. [CrossRef] [PubMed]
15. Gicquel, C. Epigenetic regulation and fetal programming. *Best Pract. Res. Clin. Endocrinol. Metab.* **2008**, *22*, 1–16. [CrossRef] [PubMed]
16. Fowden, A.L.; Giussani, D.A.; Forhead, A.J. Intrauterine Programming of Physiological Systems: Causes and Consequences. *Physiology* **2006**, *21*, 29. [CrossRef] [PubMed]

17. Grewal, J.; Grantz, K.L.; Zhang, C.; Sciscione, A.; Wing, D.A.; Grobman, W.A.; Newman, R.B.; Wapner, R.; D'Alton, M.E.; Skupski, D.; et al. Cohort Profile: NICHD Fetal Growth Studies-Singletons and Twins. *Int. J. Epidemiol.* **2017**, *47*, 25–251. [CrossRef] [PubMed]
18. Institute of Medicine (US) Committee to Review Dietary Reference Intakes for Vitamin D and Calcium. Overview of Vitamin D. In *Dietary Reference Intakes for Calcium and Vitamin D*; Ross, A., Taylor, C., Yaktine, A., Eds.; National Academies Press: Washington, DC, USA, 2011.
19. Oken, E.; Kleinman, K.P.; Rich-Edwards, J.; Gillman, M.W. A nearly continuous measure of birth weight for gestational age using a United States national reference. *BMC Pediatr.* **2003**, *3*, 6. [CrossRef] [PubMed]
20. Ulijaszek, S.J.; Kerr, D.A. Anthropometric measurement error and the assessment of nutritional status. *Br. J. Nutr.* **1999**, *82*, 165–177. [CrossRef] [PubMed]
21. Johnson, T.S.; Engstrom, J.L.; Gelhar, D.K. Intra- and interexaminer reliability of anthropometric measurements of term infants. *J. Pediatr. Gastroenterol. Nutr.* **1997**, *24*, 497–505. [CrossRef] [PubMed]
22. De Onis, M.; Onyango, A.W.; Van Den Broeck, J.; Chumlea, C.W.; Martorell, R. Measurement and standardization protocols for anthropometry used in the construction of a new international growth reference. *Food Nutr. Bull.* **2004**, *25* (Suppl. 1), S27–S36. [CrossRef] [PubMed]
23. Zhang, C.; Hediger, M.L.; Albert, P.S.; Grewal, J. Association of Maternal Obesity with Longitudinal Ultrasonographic Measures of Fetal Growth: Findings from the NICHD Fetal Growth Studies-Singletons. *JAMA Pediatr.* **2018**, *172*, 24. [CrossRef] [PubMed]
24. Chasan-Taber, L.; Schmidt, M.D.; Roberts, D.E.; Hosmer, D.; Markenson, G.; Freedson, P.S. Development and validation of a Pregnancy Physical Activity Questionnaire. *Med. Sci. Sports Exer.* **2004**, *36*, 1750–1760. [CrossRef]
25. Millen, A.E.; Pettinger, M.; Freudenheim, J.L.; Langer, R.D.; Rosenberg, C.A.; Mossavar-Rahmani, Y.; Duffy, C.M.; Lane, D.S.; Mctiernan, A.; Kuller, L.H.; et al. Incident invasive breast cancer, geographic location of residence, and reported average time spent outside. *Cancer Epidemiol. Biomark. Prev.* **2009**, *18*, 495–507. [CrossRef] [PubMed]
26. Samuelsen, S.O. A psudolikelihood approach to analysis of nested case-control studies. *Biometrika* **1997**, *84*, 379–394. [CrossRef]
27. Hinkle, S.N.; Rawal, S.; Liu, D.; Chen, J.; Tsai, M.; Zhang, C. Maternal Adipokines Longitudinally Measured Across Pregnancy and their Associations with Neonatal Size, Length, and Adiposity. *Int. J. Obes.* **2018**, in press.
28. Bischoff-Ferrari, H.A.; Giovannucci, E.; Willett, W.C.; Dietrich, T.; Dawson-Hughes, B. Estimation of optimal serum concentrations of 25-hydroxyvitamin D for multiple health outcomes. *Am. J. Clin. Nutr.* **2006**, *84*, 18–28. [CrossRef] [PubMed]
29. Leffelaar, E.R.; Vrijkotte, T.G.M.; Van Eijsden, M. Maternal early pregnancy vitamin D status in relation to fetal and neonatal growth: Results of the multi-ethnic Amsterdam Born Children and their Development cohort. *Br. J. Nutr.* **2010**, *104*, 108–117. [CrossRef] [PubMed]
30. Gernand, A.D.; Simhan, H.N.; Klebanoff, M.A.; Bodnar, L.M. Maternal serum 25-hydroxyvitamin D and measures of newborn and placental weight in a U.S. multicenter cohort study. *J. Clin. Endocrinol. Metab.* **2013**, *98*, 398–404. [CrossRef] [PubMed]
31. Miliku, K.; Vinkhuyzen, A.; Blanken, L.M.; Mcgrath, J.J.; Eyles, D.W.; Burne, T.H.; Hofman, A.; Tiemeier, H.; Steegers, E.A.; Gaillard, R.; et al. Maternal vitamin D concentrations during pregnancy, fetal growth patterns, and risks of adverse birth outcomes. *Am. J. Clin. Nutr.* **2016**, *103*, 1514–1522. [CrossRef] [PubMed]
32. Bowyer, L.; Catling-Paull, C.; Diamond, T.; Homer, C.; Davis, G.; Craig, M.E. Vitamin D, PTH and calcium levels in pregnant women and their neonates. *Clin. Endocrinol.* **2009**, *70*, 372–377. [CrossRef] [PubMed]
33. Bodnar, L.M.; Catov, J.M.; Zmuda, J.M.; Cooper, M.E.; Parrott, M.S.; Roberts, J.M.; Marazita, M.L.; Simhan, H.N. Maternal serum 25-hydroxyvitamin D concentrations are associated with small-for-gestational age births in white women. *J. Nutr.* **2010**, *140*, 999–1006. [CrossRef] [PubMed]
34. The American College of Obstetricians and Gynecologists. Prenatal Development: How the Baby Grows During Pregnancy. 2015. Available online: https://www.acog.org/Patients/FAQs/Prenatal-Development-How-Your-Baby-Grows-During-Pregnancy (accessed on 1 August 2017).
35. Hacker, A.N.; Fung, E.B.; King, J.C. Role of calcium during pregnancy: Maternal and fetal needs. *Nutr. Rev.* **2012**, *70*, 397–409. [CrossRef] [PubMed]

Nutrients **2018**, *10*, 1631

36. Kovacs, C.S. Bone development and mineral homeostasis in the fetus and neonate: Roles of the calciotropic and phosphotropic hormones. *Physiol. Rev.* **2014**, *94*, 1143–1218. [CrossRef] [PubMed]
37. Young, B.E.; Mcnanley, T.J.; Cooper, E.M.; Mcintyre, A.W.; Witter, F.; Harris, Z.L.; O'brien, K.O. Maternal vitamin D status and calcium intake interact to affect fetal skeletal growth in utero in pregnant adolescents. *Am. J. Clin. Nutr.* **2012**, *95*, 1103–1112. [CrossRef] [PubMed]
38. Pittas, A.G.; Dawson-Hughes, B.; Li, T.; Van Dam, R.M.; Willett, W.C.; Manson, J.E.; Hu, F.B. Vitamin D and Calcium Intake in Relation to Type 2 Diabetes in Women. *Diabetes Care* **2006**, *29*, 650–656. [CrossRef] [PubMed]
39. Wortsman, J.; Matsuoka, L.Y.; Chen, T.C.; Lu, Z.; Holick, M.F. Decreased bioavailability of vitamin D in obesity. *Am. J. Clin. Nutr.* **2000**, *72*, 690–693. [CrossRef] [PubMed]
40. Drincic, A.T.; Armas, L.A.; Van Diest, E.E.; Heaney, R.P. Volumetric dilution, rather than sequestration best explains the low vitamin D status of obesity. *Obesity (Silver Spring)* **2012**, *20*, 1444–1448. [CrossRef] [PubMed]
41. Headen, I.; Cohen, A.K.; Mujahid, M.; Abrams, B. The accuracy of self-reported pregnancy-related weight: A systematic review. *Obes. Rev.* **2017**, *18*, 350–369. [CrossRef] [PubMed]

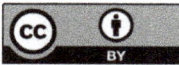

nutrients

MDPI

Article

The Impact of Maternal Pre-Pregnancy Body Weight and Gestational Diabetes on Markers of Folate Metabolism in the Placenta

Jole Martino [1,2], Maria Teresa Segura [2], Luz García-Valdés [2], M C. Padilla [3], Ricardo Rueda [4], Harry J. McArdle [5], Helen Budge [1], Michael E. Symonds [1,6,*] and Cristina Campoy [2]

[1] Early Life Research Unit, Division of Child Health and Obstetrics and Gynaecology, Nottingham NG7 2UH, UK; jolemartino78@gmail.com (J.M.); helen.budge@nottingham.ac.uk (H.B.)
[2] EURISTIKOS Excellence Centre for Paediatric Research, University of Granada, 18071 Granada, Spain; msegura@ugr.es (M.T.S.); luzgarciavaldes@hotmail.com (L.G.-V.); ccampoy@ugr.es (C.C.)
[3] Department of Obstetrics and Gynaecology, University of Granada, 18071 Granada, Spain; carmenpadvin@gmail.com
[4] Abbott Nutrition, 18004 Granada, Spain; ricardo.rueda@abbott.com
[5] The Rowett Institute of Nutrition and Health, University of Aberdeen, Aberdeen AB24 3FX UK; h.mcardle@abdn.ac.uk
[6] Nottingham Digestive Disease Centre, Biomedical Research Unit, School of Medicine, University of Nottingham, Nottingham NG7 2UH, UK
* Correspondence: michael.symonds@nottingham.ac.uk; Tel.: +44-11-5823-0625; Fax: +44-11-5823-0627

Received: 18 October 2018; Accepted: 10 November 2018; Published: 13 November 2018

check for updates

Abstract: Dietary methyl donors, including folate, may modify the placenta and size at birth but the influence of maternal body weight has not been widely investigated. We therefore examined whether maternal or fetal folate status, together with indices of placental folate transport, were modulated by either maternal pre-pregnancy body mass index (BMI i.e., overweight: $25 \le BMI < 30$ or obesity: $BMI \ge 30 \ kg/m^2$) and/or gestational diabetes mellitus (GD). We utilised a sub-sample of 135 pregnant women participating in the Spanish PREOBE survey for our analysis (i.e., 59 healthy normal weight, 29 overweight, 22 obese and 25 GD). They were blood sampled at 34 weeks gestation, and, at delivery, when a placental sample was taken together with maternal and cord blood. Placental gene expression of folate transporters and DNA methyltransferases (DNMT) were all measured. Folate plasma concentrations were determined with an electro-chemiluminescence immunoassay. Food diaries indicated that folate intake was unaffected by BMI or GD and, although all women maintained normal folate concentrations (i.e., 5–16 ng/mL), higher BMIs were associated with reduced maternal folate concentrations at delivery. Umbilical cord folate was not different, reflecting an increased concentration gradient between the mother and her fetus. Placental mRNA abundance for the folate receptor alpha (*FOLR1*) was reduced with obesity, whilst *DNMT1* was increased with raised BMI, responses that were unaffected by GD. Multi-regression analysis to determine the best predictors for placental *FOLR1* indicated that pre-gestational BMI had the greatest influence. In conclusion, the placenta's capacity to maintain fetal folate supply was not compromised by either obesity or GD.

Keywords: body mass index; gestational diabetes; placenta; folic acid

1. Introduction

Folate is an essential cofactor in metabolic pathways that influence DNA methylation patterns, DNA synthesis and cell proliferation [1,2]. It is crucial to the 1-carbon cycle where it acts as a transporter of CH3 and the single carbon donor in one carbon metabolism [3]. Limited dietary availability can contribute to abnormal DNA methylation patterns in mice [4] and, thus, potentially to developmental programming [5]. Fortification of the diet with folic acid has been adopted by many countries to ensure that dietary intake is rarely limited, particularly during pregnancy, in order to prevent neural tube defects when folate requirements can increase because of increased rates of cell division and growth, especially during embryo development [6,7]. Indeed, it is now recommended that, during pregnancy, there should be no upper limit on dietary intake [8]. Pregnant women with high body mass index (BMI) and gestational diabetes (GD) can have inadequate dietary intakes of folate [9–11] and lower folate concentrations [12,13]. This could contribute to some of the adverse neonatal outcomes associated with maternal obesity [14], including greater risks of preterm deliveries, neural tube defects and low birth weight [15–17].

Cellular uptake of folate is mediated by specific transport mechanisms in the placenta, which include the folate receptor alpha (FOLR1), proton coupled folate transporter (PCFT), and folate carrier (RFC) [18,19]. Of these mechanisms, FOLR1 appears to be the most important, at least as far as preterm births are concerned [20]. Folate is bound to the FOLR1 on the maternal side of the placenta and then transported to the fetal circulation by endocytosis/exocytosis [21]. The impact of maternal obesity on the potential capacity of the placenta to modulate folate status acting through FOLR1 has not been examined extensively in humans. One study in women in Texas found that when gestational weight gain was similar in obese and non-obese women, fetal serum folate concentrations and placental folate transport activity were unaffected [22].

The present study, was designed to explore the effects of a raised maternal pre-pregnancy BMI and/or gestational diabetes on markers of folate placental transport and metabolism, taking into account folic acid status and intake under these different maternal metabolic environments. We hypothesised that as folate has a crucial role in providing methyl donors [3], it can influence gene expression for DNA methyltransferases (DNMT1) and DNMT3A [4]. We therefore examined whether potential changes in placental folate transport resulting from high maternal BMI and/or GD, would modulate gene expression of *DNMT*. Our study was conducted in pregnant women from Spain recruited as part of the PREOBE study in which we have previously shown that placental expression of genes involved in energy sensing and oxidative stress are sensitive to maternal obesity (i.e., BMI $\geq$ 30 kg/m^2) and GD [23].

2. Materials and Methods

2.1. Participants

The participants were part of a longitudinal study on the influence of body composition by maternal genetics and nutrition (PREOBE Excellence Project: P06-CTS-02341) undertaken between 2007 and 2010 and registered with www.ClinicalTrials.gov, (NCT01634464) [24–26] for which full details have already been published (and are summarised in Table 1 [23]). It was conducted according to the guidelines in the Declaration of Helsinki and all experimental procedures were approved by the Ethics Committees for Granada University, San Cecilio University Hospital and the University of Nottingham. Witnessed, written informed consent was obtained from all participants before their study inclusion and they were assured of anonymity. Anthropometric assessments of mothers and newborns were undertaken following the standards established by the Spanish Society of Gynaecology and Obstetrics, the Fetal Foundation and the Spanish Association of Paediatrics. Gestational Diabetes was diagnosed according to the Spanish consensus protocol established by the *Grupo Español de Diabetes y Embarazo (GEDE) of the* Gynecology and Obstetricians Society, followed by Andalusian pregnant women general practitioners [27]. The O'Sullivan test was performed on all pregnant women between 24–28 weeks of pregnancy, as screening for gestational diabetes. If glucose was $\geq$140 mg/dL an oral glucose tolerance test (OGTT) with 100 g of glucose loading was performed. Gestational diabetes was diagnosed if two or more glucose values met or exceeded the following values fasting <105 mg/dL, one hour <190 mg/dL, two hours <165 mg/dL, three hours <145 mg/dL. Women with plasma glucose ≥ 200 mg/dL after O'Sullivan test were diagnosed of gestational diabetes and OGTT was not performed. The O'Sullivan screening test was also performed in the first trimester in high risk pregnant women (maternal age >35 years; BMI > 30 kg/m^2, previous gestational diabetes or other glucose metabolic alterations, previous obstetric results with an indication of undiagnosed gestational diabetes (e.g., *foetal macrosomy*), family history of diabetes mellitus, ethnic risk groups (Afroamericans, Asiatic-Americans, Hispanic, Indio-Americans))

Table 1. Summary of maternal age, body and birth weights of all participants.

	N (*n* = 59)	OW (*n* = 29)	O (*n* = 22)	GDN (*n* = 14)	GDO (*n* = 11)
Maternal characteristics					
Age at delivery (years)	30.4 ± 4.5	30.9 ± 7.2	29.0 ± 4.7	33.1 ± 4.1 *	34.7 ± 4.3 **
Height (cm)	162.9 ± 5.7	162.5 ± 6.4	162.7 ± 6.2	159.3 ± 3.9	160.5 ± 6.0
Pre pregnancy BMI (kg/m^2)	21.8 ± 1.8	27.8 ± 2.2 ***	32.5 ± 2.6 ***	22.4 ± 1.8	35.5 ± 4.9 ***
BMI at 34 weeks (kg/m^2)	26.6 ± 2.6	31.3 ± 2.4 ***	35.4 ± 2.4 ***	25.9 ± 2.6	36.4 ± 4.1 ***
GWG 0–34 weeks (kg)	12.6 ± 4.3	9.9 ± 4.6 **	7.3 ± 5.1 ***	9.0 ± 5.6 **	2.2 ± 7.8 ***
Preterm (<37 gestational weeks) (*n*)	2 (3%)	1 (3%)	2 (9%).	1 (14%)	4 (27%) *
Male newborn (%)	53	40	62	57	73
Number of caesarean section (%)	12	26	38	25	50
Number on supplements $^+$	45	26	22	12	9
Infant characteristics					
Newborn weight (g)	3292 ± 410	3230 ± 587	3454 ± 549	3374 ± 402	3415 ± 549
Placental weight (g)	469 ± 120	495 ± 135	531 ± 114 *	498 ± 134	476 ± 93
Placental: birth weight ratio	0.14 ± 0.03	0.16 ± 0.05	0.16 ± 0.04	0.15 ± 0.04	0.14 ± 0.02
Gestational age (weeks)	39.2 ± 1.0	39.4 ± 1.6	39.3 ± 1.7	39.3 ± 1.3	38.8 ± 1.3

Pre: pregestational; BMI: body mass index; GWG: gestational weight gain during the first 34 gestational weeks based on 2009 IOM guidelines for each category [28]. $^+$ reported taking folate and iodine supplements at 24th week of gestation. Values are means ± SD or categorical data as appropriate; n: number of women per group; gw: weeks of gestational. Statistical differences: * $p < 0.05$, ** $p < 0.01$, *** $p < 0.001$ compared to normal w eight group (Chi-square test or t-independent test for continuous variables; chi-square test for categorical variables). Based on their pre-pregnancy weights they were classified as being of normal weight (N), overweight (OW), obese (O), gestational diabetic, normal weight (GDN) or gestational diabetic, obese (GDO) pregnant women (Martino et al., 2016) [23].

As shown in Table 1, the subpopulation of 135 participants whose placentas underwent molecular analysis in Nottingham, for which a majority that gave birth at full term i.e., c. 39 weeks [23], with the exception of GDO for which 50% underwent caesarean section delivery. The number of participants per group were, therefore, 59 normal weight women ($18 \leq$ pre-pregnancy BMI < 25 kg/m^2 (N)), 29 overweight women ($25 \leq$ BMI < 30 kg/m^2 (OW)) and 22 obese women (BMI $\geq$ 30 kg/m^2 (O)). Furthermore, the 25 mothers with GD were subsequently classified according to their BMI as normal weight GD (pre-pregnancy BMI < 25 kg/m^2 (GDN), *n* = 14) and as obese GD (pre-pregnancy BMI $\geq$ 30 kg/m^2 (GDO), *n* = 11). There were no effects of the sex of the baby, route of delivery or gestational age on any of the measurements reported in this study.

2.2. Maternal Nutrient Intake

Information about maternal nutrient intake was collected during late gestation (34–40 weeks) using standardised 7 day dietary records given to the participants during the second visit (34th gestational week). Each participant was given verbal and written instructions by the investigator on how to record food and drinks consumed during the 7 day recording period and a booklet of common food items and mixed dishes to facilitate estimation of portion sizes. Around the time of delivery, food records were reviewed with each mother by a nutritionist for completeness and accuracy of food description and portion sizes. Nutritional data were analysed for nutrient intake by using a nutritional software program (CESNID 1.0: Barcelona University, Spain) based on validated Spanish food tables ("*Tablas de composición de alimentos del CESNID*") [29] and took account of those products fortified with folic acid.

2.3. Collection and Analysis of Blood Samples

Maternal venous blood was collected at 34 weeks of gestation and during labour (N: $n = 59$; OW: $n = 29$; O: $n = 22$; GDN: $n = 14$; GDO: $n = 11$). Umbilical venous blood samples (N: $n = 33$; OW: $n = 15$; O: $n = 12$; GDN: $n = 7$; GDO: $n = 7$) were collected within 30 min after placental delivery from a double-clamped section of umbilical cord. EDTA and serum collection tubes were used (Vacutainer® Refs: 368857 and 367953) for haematological assessment and biochemical analyses respectively. There were no differences in any of the measurements performed on the placenta between those women from whom blood was sampled and those in whom this could not be achieved e.g., born at a time when sampling could not be undertaken.

Blood samples for serum preparation were held at 4 °C for 15 min to allow blood clotting, centrifuged at 3500 rpm for 10 min at 4 °C, and the serum fraction transferred into sterile tubes. Samples were stored at 4 °C for same-day analyses or at −80 °C for further analysis. Serum folate was determined by an electro-chemiluminescence immunoassay with the automatic analyser Elecsys 2010, and the analytical kit No. E170 (Roche, Neuilly sur Seine, France).

2.4. Collection of Placenta Samples

Placenta samples from all participants were collected and weighed immediately after delivery as previously published [23]. Visual inspection of the placenta for necrosis or any other abnormality was undertaken by experienced clinicians. A representative $0.5 \times 0.5 \times 0.5$ cm (200 mg) sample was excised from the middle of the radius (distance between the insertion of the umbilical cord and the periphery) of each placenta, rinsed twice with saline solution (0.9% NaCl) and immediately placed into sterile 1.5 mL microtubes (Greiner Bio One, Monroe, NC, USA) containing RNAlater solution (Qiagen Ltd., Crawley, UK). All samples were frozen under RNase free conditions using liquid nitrogen before storage at −80 °C for later analysis in Nottingham.

2.5. Laboratory Analysis

Total RNA was extracted from 100 mg of maternal placenta tissue using 200 µL of chloroform per 1 mL of TRI reagent solution (Sigma Chemical Co., Poole, UK) and RNeasy extraction kit (Qiagen Ltd., Crawley, UK) as previously published [23]. RNA quality was assessed by gel electropheresis. Two µg RNA was used to generate 20 µL cDNA using High Capacity RNA-to-cDNA kit (Applied Biosystems, Foster City, CA, USA). Negative control RT samples lacking Enzyme Mix (-RT) were included for each sample. Real-time PCR using 15 µL of reactions consisting of 4.5 µL diluted 1:10 cDNA, 3.0 µL (final concentration of 250 nM) gene specific primers (Table 2, Sigma-Aldrich, St. Louis, MO, USA), and 7.5 µL of SYBR Green mastermix (Thermo Scientific, ABgene Ltd., Epson, UK) were performed. Duplicate samples were run for 40 cycles with negative controls in 96-well plates using the Techne Quantica Thermocycler (Techne Inc., Barloword Scientific, Stone, UK). Ten-fold serial dilutions of cDNA for each gene were used to generate standard curve analysis and only experiments with R^2 > 0.985 were included. CT measurements, calculated by $2^{-\Delta Ct}$ method [30], were used for mRNA expression. A range of housekeeping genes were used including *ACT8*, *18S* and *B2M*, for which 18S ribosomal RNA was used as the optimal housekeeping gene for data normalisation, as previously published [23]. It was the most stable housekeeping examined (i.e., N: 0.37 ± 0.08; OW 0.70 ± 0.28; OB 0.56 ± 0.11; GDL 0.75 ± 0.14; GDO 0.13 ± 0.02 a.u.) and the use of other reference genes made no difference to the results.

Table 2. Summary of primers used together with qPCR product and conditions.

Target Gene	Forward Primer Sequence	Reverse Primer Sequence	Product Size (bp)	Temp (°C)
FOLR1	CACTCCCTGCCTGTCTCC	TCTGCTCTGCTCTACACTCC	80	59
PCFT (SLC46A1)	ATGCAGCTTTCTGCTTTGGT	GGAGCCACATAGAGCTGGAC	100	60
RFC (SLC19A1)	CAGCATCTGGCTGTGCTATG	TGATGGTCTTGACGATGGTG	161	59
MTHFR	TCCCGTCAGCTTCATGTTCT	TGTCGTGGATGTACTGGATGA	116	59
DNMT1	TTCTTCGCAGAGCAAATTGA	CGTCATCTGCCTCCTTCATGG	210	57
DNMT3A	AAGCCTCAAGAGCAGTGGAA	AAGCAGACCTTTAGCCACGA	190	59

FOLR1: folate receptor alpha; *PCFT*: proton coupled folate transporter; *RFC*: reduced folate carrier; *MTHFR*: methylenetetrahydrofolate reductase; *DNMT1*: DNA methyl transferase-1; *DNMT3A*: DNA methyl transferase-3 alpha. bp, base pairs.

2.6. Statistical Analysis

All statistical evaluations were performed by using IBM SPSS v20.0 statistical software for Windows (IBM Corp., Armonk, NY, USA). To assess the data for normality, a Kolmogorov–Smirnov test was performed, where *p* values >0.05 indicated that the data were normally distributed. Thereafter, appropriate parametric, or non-parametric, tests were used to analyse the effects of maternal overweight and obesity as follows: (1) comparisons of blood folate concentration at each sampling age between comparable groups (i.e., N vs. OW, or O, or GDN; GDN vs. GDO) were made by independent *t*-test; whilst (2) differences in gene expression were determined by using Mann-Whitney test. Categorical data were analysed using Chi-square test of independence. Continuous data (i.e., gene expression and folate concentrations) presented are expressed as means with their standard errors (SEM), with *p* values < 0.05 deemed to represent statistical significance. For all analyses undertaken, there was no effect of foetal sex or route of delivery.

Association between continuous variables were also assessed using multiple linear regression analysis. It included the following three models: The first was adjusted for the a priori confounder of pre-gestational BMI; the second, for both BMI and maternal glucose at 34 weeks of gestation and the third for BMI, maternal glucose and folate at 34 weeks gestation.

3. Results

Maternal Folate Status and Adaptations within the Placenta

Amongst those participants for whom placental analysis was undertaken and who reported daily intakes of folate (400 µg dietary folate equivalents/day) and iodine supplements at 24th week of pregnancy, there were no differences in folate or vitamin B12 consumption between groups (Table 3). Folate concentrations in all participants in the present study were within the normal range (6–20 ng/mL) with no evidence of folate deficiency (defined as <5 ng/mL: Figure 1) [7]. GDN women exhibited the highest serum folate concentrations at 34 gestational weeks compared to the normal weight group (Figure 1). This could reflect dietary and related advice given to this sub-group, in which mean folate and vitamin B12 intakes were also highest (Table 3). There was no significant effect of taking folate supplements in late gestation on maternal folate concentrations at 40 weeks of gestation. A marked decrease in folate concentrations in late pregnancy was observed in both OW and O women (Figure 1). Cord blood folate concentrations were not different between groups, reflecting an increased difference between maternal folate at 40 gestational weeks and umbilical cord folate with raised maternal BMI (i.e., Δ folate–N: 5.80 $\pm$ 0.81; OW: 7.66 $\pm$ 0.82; O: 9.01 $\pm$ 0.90 ng/mL ($p < 0.05$)). There was also a positive correlation between maternal and newborn plasma folate in the N ($r^2 = 0.38$; $p < 0.0001$) and GDN ($r^2 = 0.81$; $p = 0.015$) groups at 34 weeks gestation and in the N ($r^2 = 0.19$; $p = 0.013$) and OW ($r^2 = 0.48$; $p = 0.006$) groups at 40 weeks gestation. No infants exhibited any spinal or neural abnormalities.

Table 3. Mean maternal 7 day dietary intake of folate and vitamin B12 between 34–40 weeks gestation for each group of women whose body weight category was defined according to their pre pregnancy BMI.

Maternal Intake (µg DFE/day)	N (*n* = 37)	OW (*n* = 15)	O (*n* = 8)	GDN (*n* = 11)	GDO (*n* = 6)
Folate	298 ± 12	258 ± 18	260 ± 46	342 ± 33	299 ± 53
Vitamin B12	5.8 ± 0.5	4.7 ± 0.5	5.3 ± 0.9	10.1 ± 4.1	5.3 ± 1.2

DEF, dietary folate equivalents. Normal weight: N; overweight: OW; obese: O, gestational diabetic, normal weight: GDN and gestational diabetic, obese: GDO. Values are means ± SD.

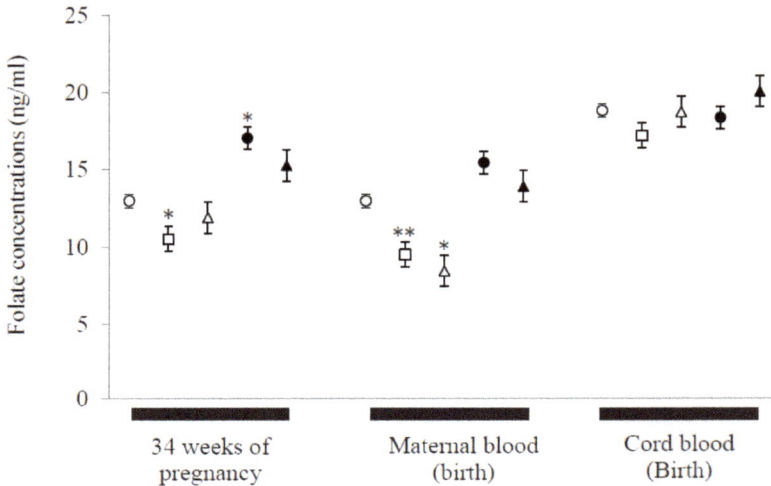

Figure 1. Effects of maternal pre-pregnancy BMI and gestational diabetes on maternal and neonatal folate serum concentrations. Maternal samples were taken at 34 weeks gestation and at term/delivery i.e., c. 39 weeks of pregnancy, neonatal samples were taken from cord blood at birth. Open circles: normal weight (N: maternal, *n* = 59; cord, *n* = 33); open squares: overweight (OW: maternal, *n* = 29; cord, *n* = 15); open triangles: obese (O: maternal, *n* = 22; cord, *n* = 12); closed circles: gestational diabetic, normal weight (GDN: maternal, *n* = 14; cord, *n* = 7); closed triangles: gestational diabetic, obese women (GDO: maternal, *n* = 11; cord, *n* = 7). Values represent means ± S.E.M. Statistical differences between groups denoted at each time point by *, ** correspond to $p < 0.05$, $p < 0.01$ respectively compared to normal weight control group (independent t test for continuous variables).

Placentas from obese women showed a significantly lower expression of *FOLR1*, a response that was unaffected by GD (Table 4). Multi-regression analysis of predictors for placental *FOLR1* gene expression, indicated that pre-pregnancy BMI had the greatest influence (Table 5), suggesting an effect present in early gestation. Gene expression of placental methylenetetrahydrofolate reductase (NAD(P)H) (*MTHFR*), the enzyme that catalyses the synthesis of 5-MTHF, did not significantly change between BMI groups, but was raised in obese women with GD (Table 4). Whilst placental *DNMT3A* gene expression was similar between groups, mean mRNA expression of *DNMT1* was higher in overweight and women (Table 4). No significant correlations were found between placental gene expression and plasma folate.

Table 4. Effects of maternal body mass index on gene expression markers of folate transport and metabolism and DNA methylation in placenta of normal weight (N), overweight (OW), obese (O), gestational diabetic, normal weight (GDN) and gestational diabetic, obese (GDO) pregnant women.

Pathway	NCBI Sequence	Target Gene	N (n = 59)	OW (n = 29)	O (n = 21)	GDN (n = 14)	GDO (n = 11)
Folate transport and metabolism	NM_016725.2	*FOLR1*	1.0 ± 0.9	0.8 ± 0.6	0.5 ± 0.3 *	0.6 ± 0.3	0.5 ± 0.3 *
	NM_080669.4	*PCFT* $^\psi$	1.0 ± 0.6	1.0 ± 0.6	1.1 ± 0.6	0.6 ± 0.7	0.8 ± 0.5
	NM_006996.2	*RFC* $^\psi$	1.0 ± 0.8	0.9 ± 0.5	1.0 ± 0.7	0.8 ± 0.5	0.7 ± 0.5
	NM_005957	*MTHFR*	1.0 ± 0.9	1.0 ± 0.9	0.8 ± 0.6	1.0 ± 0.7	1.5 ± 0.7 *
DNA methylation	NM_001130823	*DNMT1*	1.0 ± 1.1	1.8 ± 1.1 **	1.5 ± 1.2	1.8 ± 1.5	0.5 ± 0.5
	NM_022552.4	*DNMT3A*	1.0 ± 0.9	1.1 ± 1.2	0.7 ± 0.5	0.9 ± 0.9	0.6 ± 0.3

Data expressed relative to housekeeping gene (ribosomal 18S RNA), normalised to the control group to give the fold change. n = women/group. Data are non-parametric and represent mean ± SD Statistical differences: * $p < 0.05$, ** $p < 0.01$ compared to normal weight group (Mann Whitney test). The abundance of genes denoted by $^\psi$ were measured in a representative selection of 20 N women as insufficient mRNA was not available for all samples. *FOLR1*: folate receptor alpha; *PCFT*: proton coupled folate transporter; *RFC*: reduced folate carrier; *MTHFR*: methylenetetrahydrofolate reductase; *DNMT1*: DNA methyl transferase-1; *DNMT3A*: DNA methyl transferase-3 alpha.

Table 5. Association between placental gene expression of folate receptor alpha (*FOLR1*) and different predictors in control, overweight and obese pregnant women with or without gestational diabetes (n = 135).

Linear Regression Model	B (95% CI)	SE B	β	p
Model 1 $^\psi$				
Maternal pre-BMI	−0.029 (−0.051, −0.007)	0.011	−0.214	0.009
Model 2 $^{\psi\psi}$				
Maternal pre-BMI	−0.032 (−0.054, −0.009)	0.011	−0.230	0.006
Maternal glucose (34 gw)	0.004 (−0.002, 0.01)	0.003	0.107	0.194
Model 3 $^{\psi\psi\psi}$				
Maternal pre-BMI	−0.033 (−0.056, −0.011)	0.012	−0.241	0.004
Maternal glucose (34 gw)	0.005 (−0.001, 0.01)	0.003	0.131	0.116
Maternal folate (34 gw)	−0.019 (−0.043, 0.005)	0.012	0.128	0.124

$^\psi$ Adjusted for the *a priori* confounders pre-pregnancy BMI; $^{\psi\psi}$ adjusted for the *a priori* confounders pre-pregnancy BMI and maternal glucose at 34 weeks of gestation (gw); $^{\psi\psi\psi}$ Adjusted for the *a priori* confounders pre-pregnancy BMI, maternal glucose at 34 gw and maternal folate at 34 gw. *B*: unstandardised beta; 95% CI: 95% Confidence intervals; *SE B*: Standard error of unstandardised beta; β: standardised beta (β).

4. Discussion

We show that although maternal folate concentrations were reduced with raised maternal pre-pregnancy BMI near to term, this was not apparent with GD, suggesting that the dietary advice provided improved folate status irrespective of any placental adaptations, as seen with obesity. In those women with raised pre-pregnancy BMI, there was no detectable reduction in cord blood folate and all infants were healthy at term. This suggests appropriate adaptation in folate transfer across the placenta, that has been suggested to include a downregulation of *FOLR1* gene expression in the placenta with obesity [19]. The results from our study support such a proposal as gene expression for the other two transporters, *PCFT* and *RFC*, were unaffected. Raised mRNA abundance of *FOLR1*, if translated to protein, and accompanied with a decline in maternal folate concentration would result in the maintenance of cord blood folate as we observed at term with obesity. Alternatively mRNA transcripts of this folate transporter could undergo further functional modifications, that modulate the placentas capacity to promote folate transport [31] and, hence, protect normal foetal folate status as seen in women from Texas, USA [22].

The negative association between raised pre-pregnancy BMI and folate status did not appear to be related to dietary inadequacy in these women unlike those described by others [9–11]. It is possible that other adaptations to a high pre-pregnancy BMI, such as hormonal changes in pregnancy and endocrine modifications, could contribute [6]. It is possible that adaptations within the maternal microbiome could impact on maternal folate status [32], as has been shown in the rat during late gestation when manipulating macronutrient intake [33]. Interestingly, obesity with GD resulted in raised placental *MTHFR* gene expression that could ultimately inhibit intracellular homocysteine release by promoting 5-MTHF synthesis [34–36]. Enhanced folate catabolism by the placenta would also limit homocysteine accumulation within the trophoblast, thereby avoiding foetal complications in women with obesity and/or GD [35,37].

As folate deficiency has been associated with increased placental S-adenosyl-methionine to S-adenosyl-homocysteine ratio [38,39] and decreased genomic DNA methylation [40–43], reduced blood folate with obesity could lower the availability of placental SAM, which is used by DNMTs to methylate DNA [2,44,45]. Changes in gene expression for *DNMT1* could be important in this regard as it transcribes the enzyme required for the maintenance of DNA methylation [46] although this was not measured in the present study. DNMT1 is also essential for cellular development [46] and our observation of raised placental gene expression with increased BMI could impact on these processes even though *DNMT3A* was unaffected. These divergent responses could reflect their contrasting roles, with DNMT3A catalysing de novo DNA methylation during early development, whilst DNMT1 is responsible for the maintenance of DNA methylation throughout all development stages [4]. The decreased maternal folate with raised pre-pregnancy BMI and higher mRNA abundance of *DNMT1* in the placenta with similar cord blood folate concentrations, could be indicative of a compensatory response in order to maintain adequate methylation status, for which no differences were found when measured in five subjects per study group [47]. Overall the relatively small sample size was utilised in our study, which might benefit from being undertaken in larger groups of women of different ethnicity. Such a broader study could be combined with a more detailed assessment of those epigenetic adaptations which remain to be clarified [48].

5. Conclusions

In conclusion, pregnancies in Spanish women with a high BMI and GD are differentially associated with changes in maternal serum folate in late gestation, which suggests a protective role by the placenta of the foetus, further supporting the need to ensure optimal dietary folate intake [8].

Author Contributions: J.M.—conducted placental analysis, performed all statistical analysis and co-drafted manuscript. M.T.S.—collected samples and patient information. L.G.-V.—collected patient information and conducted blood sample analysis. M.C.P.—collected samples and patient information. R.R.—co-formulated the research question, co-supervised the project and edited the manuscript. H.J.M.—co-supervised the project and edited the manuscript. H.B.—co-supervised the project and edited the manuscript. M.E.S.—co-supervised the project and co-drafted the manuscript. C.C.—co-formulated the research question, led the project and edited the manuscript.

Funding: The Spanish Ministry of Innovation and Science, Junta de Andalucía (Ref. N°: P06-CTS-0234), Spanish Ministry of Economy and Competitiveness (Grant no. BFU2012-40254-C03-01); Abbott Nutrition, Spain; The Nottingham Respiratory Biomedical Research Unit, and the Nottingham University Hospitals Charity. This work was also supported by the Medical Research Council (Grant numbers G0800129-1 and 1G0600310).

Acknowledgments: The authors wish to thank participants and clinical staff for their support of this study.

Conflicts of Interest: The authors declare no conflicts of interest.

References

1. Portela, A.; Esteller, M. Epigenetic modifications and human disease. *Nat. Biotechnol.* **2010**, *28*, 1057–1068. [CrossRef] [PubMed]
2. Filiberto, A.C.; Maccani, M.A.; Koestler, D.C.; Wilhelm-Benartzi, C.; Avissar-Whiting, M.; Banister, C.E.; Gagne, L.A.; Marsit, C.J. Birthweight is associated with DNA promoter methylation of the glucocorticoid receptor in human placenta. *Epigenetics* **2011**, *6*, 566–572. [CrossRef] [PubMed]

3. Kim, J.M.; Hong, K.; Lee, J.H.; Lee, S.; Chang, N. Effect of folate deficiency on placental DNA methylation in hyperhomocysteinemic rats. *J. Nutr. Biochem.* **2009**, *20*, 172–176. [CrossRef] [PubMed]
4. Ding, Y.B.; He, J.L.; Liu, X.Q.; Chen, X.M.; Long, C.L.; Wang, Y.X. Expression of DNA methyltransferases in the mouse uterus during early pregnancy and susceptibility to dietary folate deficiency. *Reproduction* **2012**, *144*, 91–100. [CrossRef] [PubMed]
5. Barres, R.; Zierath, J.R. DNA methylation in metabolic disorders. *Am. J. Clin. Nutr.* **2011**, *93*, 897S–900S. [CrossRef] [PubMed]
6. Kim, H.; Hwang, J.Y.; Kim, K.N.; Ha, E.H.; Park, H.; Ha, M.; Lee, K.Y.; Hong, Y.C.; Tamura, T.; Chang, N. Relationship between body-mass index and serum folate concentrations in pregnant women. *Eur. J. Clin. Nutr.* **2012**, *66*, 136–138. [CrossRef] [PubMed]
7. Serum and Red Blood Cell Folate Concentrations for Assessing Folate Status in Populations. Available online: http://apps.who.int/iris/bitstream/10665/75584/1/WHO_NMH_NHD_EPG_12.1_eng.pdf (accessed on 1 October 2016).
8. Wald, N.J.; Morris, J.K.; Blakemore, C. Public health failure in the prevention of neural tube defects: Time to abandon the tolerable upper intake level of folate. *Pub. Health Rev.* **2018**, *39*, 2. [CrossRef] [PubMed]
9. Guelinckx, I.; Devlieger, R.; Beckers, K.; Vansant, G. Maternal obesity: Pregnancy complications, gestational weight gain and nutrition. *Obes. Rev.* **2008**, *9*, 140–150. [CrossRef] [PubMed]
10. Moran, L.J.; Sui, Z.; Cramp, C.S.; Dodd, J.M. A decrease in diet quality occurs during pregnancy in overweight and obese women which is maintained post-partum. *Int. J. Obes.* **2012**, *37*, 704–711. [CrossRef] [PubMed]
11. Rifas-Shiman, S.L.; Rich-Edwards, J.W.; Kleinman, K.P.; Oken, E.; Gillman, M.W. Dietary Quality during Pregnancy Varies by Maternal Characteristics in Project Viva: A US Cohort. *J. Am. Diet. Assoc.* **2009**, *109*, 1004–1011. [CrossRef] [PubMed]
12. Mojtabai, R. Body mass index and serum folate in childbearing age women. *Eur. J. Epidemiol.* **2004**, *19*, 1029–1036. [CrossRef] [PubMed]
13. Da Silva, V.R.; Hausman, D.B.; Kauwell, G.P.; Sokolow, A.; Tackett, R.L.; Rathbun, S.L.; Bailey, L.B. Obesity affects short-term folate pharmacokinetics in women of childbearing age. *Int. J. Obes.* **2013**, *37*, 1608–1610. [CrossRef] [PubMed]
14. Ray, J.G.; Wyatt, P.R.; Vermeulen, M.J.; Meier, C.; Cole, D.E. Greater maternal weight and the ongoing risk of neural tube defects after folic acid flour fortification. *Obstet. Gynecol.* **2005**, *105*, 261–265. [CrossRef] [PubMed]
15. Eichholzer, M.; Tonz, O.; Zimmermann, R. Folic acid: A public-health challenge. *Lancet* **2006**, *367*, 1352–1361. [CrossRef]
16. Oyama, K.; Sugimura, Y.; Murase, T.; Uchida, A.; Hayasaka, S.; Oiso, Y.; Murata, Y. Folic acid prevents congenital malformations in the offspring of diabetic mice. *Endocr. J.* **2009**, *56*, 29–37. [CrossRef] [PubMed]
17. Pickell, L.; Li, D.Q.; Brown, K.; Mikael, L.G.; Wang, X.L.; Wu, Q.; Luo, L.; Jerome-Majewska, L.; Rozen, R. Methylenetetrahydrofolate Reductase Deficiency and Low Dietary Folate Increase Embryonic Delay and Placental Abnormalities in Mice. *Birth Defects Res. A Clin. Mol. Teratol.* **2009**, *85*, 531–541. [CrossRef] [PubMed]
18. Antony, A.C. In utero physiology: Role of folic acid in nutrient delivery and fetal development. *Am. J. Clin. Nutr.* **2007**, *85*, 598S–603S. [CrossRef] [PubMed]
19. Solanky, N.; Jimenez, A.R.; D'Souza, S.W.; Sibley, C.P.; Glazier, J.D. Expression of folate transporters in human placenta and implications for homocysteine metabolism. *Placenta* **2010**, *31*, 134–143. [CrossRef] [PubMed]
20. Castano, E.; Caviedes, L.; Hirsch, S.; Llanos, M.; Iniguez, G.; Ronco, A.M. Folate Transporters in Placentas from Preterm Newborns and Their Relation to Cord Blood Folate and Vitamin B12 Levels. *PLoS ONE* **2017**, *12*, e0170389. [CrossRef] [PubMed]
21. Solanky, N.; Jimenez, A.R.; D'Souza, S.W.; Sibley, C.P.; Glazier, J.D. Folate Transporters in First Trimester and Term Human Placenta. *Reprod. Sci.* **2009**, *16*, 81a–82a.
22. Carter, M.F.; Powell, T.L.; Li, C.; Myatt, L.; Dudley, D.; Nathanielsz, P.; Jansson, T. Fetal serum folate concentrations and placental folate transport in obese women. *Am. J. Obstet. Gynecol.* **2011**. [CrossRef] [PubMed]
23. Martino, J.; Sebert, S.; Segura, M.T.; Garcia-Valdes, L.; Florido, J.; Padilla, M.C.; Marcos, A.; Rueda, R.; McArdle, H.J.; Budge, H.; et al. Maternal body weight and gestational diabetes differentially influence placental and pregnancy outcomes. *J. Clin. Endocrinol. Metab.* **2016**, *101*, 59–68. [CrossRef] [PubMed]

24. Torres-Espinola, F.J.; Berglund, S.K.; Garcia-Valdes, L.M.; Segura, M.T.; Jerez, A.; Campos, D.; Moreno-Torres, R.; Rueda, R.; Catena, A.; Perez-Garcia, M.; et al. Maternal obesity, overweight and gestational diabetes affect the offspring neurodevelopment at 6 and 18 months of age—A follow up from the PREOBE cohort. *PLoS ONE* **2015**, *10*, e0133010. [CrossRef] [PubMed]

25. Garcia-Valdes, L.; Campoy, C.; Hayes, H.; Florido, J.; Rusanova, I.; Miranda, M.T.; McArdle, H.J. The impact of maternal obesity on iron status, placental transferrin receptor expression and hepcidin expression in human pregnancy. *Int. J. Obes.* **2015**, *39*, 571–578. [CrossRef] [PubMed]

26. Berglund, S.K.; Garcia-Valdes, L.; Torres-Espinola, F.J.; Segura, M.T.; Martinez-Zaldivar, C.; Aguilar, M.J.; Agil, A.; Lorente, J.A.; Florido, J.; Padilla, C.; et al. Maternal, fetal and perinatal alterations associated with obesity, overweight and gestational diabetes: An observational cohort study (PREOBE). *BMC Public Health* **2016**, *16*, 207. [CrossRef] [PubMed]

27. Documento, C.d. Asistencia a la gestante con diabetes. Guía de práctica clínica actualizada en 2014 Grupo Español de Diabetes y Embarazo (GEDE). *Av. Diabetol.* **2015**, *31*, 45–59.

28. Rasmussen, K.M.; Yaktine, A.L. *Weight gain during pregnancy: Reexamining the guidelines*; The National Academies Press: Washington, DC, USA, 2009.

29. Casas-Agustench, P.; Lopez-Uriarte, P.; Bullo, M.; Ros, E.; Gomez-Flores, A.; Salas-Salvado, J. Acute effects of three high-fat meals with different fat saturations on energy expenditure, substrate oxidation and satiety. *Clin. Nutr.* **2009**, *28*, 39–45. [CrossRef] [PubMed]

30. Livak, K.J.; Schmittgen, T.D. Analysis of relative gene expression data using real-time quantitative PCR and the 2(T)(-Delta Delta C) method. *Methods* **2001**, *25*, 402–408. [CrossRef] [PubMed]

31. Caviedes, L.; Iñiguez, G.; Hidalgo, P.; Castro, J.J.; Castaño, E.; Llanos, M.; Hirsch, S.; Ronco, A.M. Relationship between folate transporters expression in human placentas at term and birth weights. *Placenta* **2016**, *38*, 24–28. [CrossRef] [PubMed]

32. Astbury, S.; Mostyn, A.; Symonds, M.E.; Bell, R.C. Nutrient availability, the microbiome, and intestinal transport during pregnancy. *Appl. Physiol. Nutr. Metab.* **2015**, *40*, 1100–1106. [CrossRef] [PubMed]

33. Astbury, S.; Song, A.; Zhou, M.; Nielsen, B.; Hoedl, A.; Willing, B.P.; Symonds, M.E.; Bell, R.C. High fructose intake during pregnancy in rats influences the maternal microbiome and gut development in the offspring. *Front. Genet.* **2018**, *9*, 203. [CrossRef] [PubMed]

34. Khong, T.Y.; Hague, W.M. The placenta in maternal hyperhomocysteinaemia. *Br. J. Obstet. Gynaecol.* **1999**, *106*, 273–278. [CrossRef] [PubMed]

35. Bergen, N.E.; Timmermans, S.; Hofman, A.; Steegers-Theunissen, R.P.; Russcher, H.; Lindemans, J.; Jaddoe, V.W.; Steegers, E.A. First trimester homocysteine and folate levels are associated with increased adverse pregnancy outcomes. *Reprod. Sci.* **2011**, *18*, S22. [CrossRef]

36. Friso, S.; Choi, S.W.; Girelli, D.; Mason, J.B.; Dolnikowski, G.G.; Bagley, P.J.; Olivieri, O.; Jacques, P.F.; Rosenberg, I.H.; Corrocher, R.; et al. A common mutation in the 5,10-methylenetetrahydrofolate reductase gene affects genomic DNA methylation through an interaction with folate status. *Proc. Natl. Acad. Sci. USA* **2002**, *99*, 5606–5611. [CrossRef] [PubMed]

37. Di Simone, N.; Maggiano, N.; Caliandro, D.; Riccardi, P.; Evangelista, A.; Carducci, B.; Caruso, A. Homocysteine induces trophoblast cell death with apoptotic features. *Biol. Reprod.* **2003**, *69*, 1129–1134. [CrossRef] [PubMed]

38. Ulrey, C.L.; Liu, L.; Andrews, L.G.; Tollefsbol, T.O. The impact of metabolism on DNA methylation. *Hum. Mol. Genet.* **2005**, *14*, R139–R147. [CrossRef] [PubMed]

39. Mikael, L.G.; Pancer, J.; Jiang, X.; Wu, Q.; Caudill, M.; Rozen, R. Low dietary folate and methylenetetrahydrofolate reductase deficiency may lead to pregnancy complications through modulation of ApoAI and IFN-gamma in spleen and placenta, and through reduction of methylation potential. *Mol. Nutr. Food Res.* **2012**. [CrossRef]

40. Cooper, W.N.; Khulan, B.; Owens, S.; Elks, C.E.; Seidel, V.; Prentice, A.M.; Belteki, G.; Ong, K.K.; Affara, N.A.; Constancia, M.; et al. DNA methylation profiling at imprinted loci after periconceptional micronutrient supplementation in humans: Results of a pilot randomized controlled trial. *FASEB J.* **2012**, *26*, 1782–1790. [CrossRef] [PubMed]

41. Rampersaud, G.C.; Kauwell, G.P.A.; Hutson, A.D.; Cerda, J.J.; Bailey, L.B. Genomic DNA methylation decreases in response to moderate folate depletion in elderly women. *Am. J. Clin. Nutr.* **2000**, *72*, 998–1003. [CrossRef] [PubMed]

42. Seki, Y.; Williams, L.; Vuguin, P.M.; Charron, M.J. Minireview: Epigenetic programming of diabetes and obesity: Animal models. *Endocrinology* **2012**, *153*, 1031–1038. [CrossRef] [PubMed]
43. Radaelli, T.; Lepercq, J.; Varastehpour, A.; Basu, S.; Catalano, P.M.; Hauguel-De Mouzon, S. Differential regulation of genes for fetoplacental lipid pathways in pregnancy with gestational and type 1 diabetes mellitus. *Am. J. Obstet. Gynecol.* **2009**. [CrossRef] [PubMed]
44. Maccani, M.A.; Marsit, C.J. Epigenetics in the Placenta. *Am. J. Reprod. Immunol.* **2009**, *62*, 78–89. [CrossRef] [PubMed]
45. Niculescu, M.D.; Zeisel, S.H. Diet, methyl donors and DNA methylation: Interactions between dietary folate, methionine and choline. *J. Nutr.* **2002**, *132*, 2333S–2335S. [CrossRef] [PubMed]
46. Robertson, K.D.; Ait-Si-Ali, S.; Yokochi, T.; Wade, P.A.; Jones, P.L.; Wolffe, A.P. DNMT1 forms a complex with Rb, E2F1 and HDAC1 and represses transcription from E2F-responsive promoters. *Nat. Genet.* **2000**, *25*, 338–342. [CrossRef] [PubMed]
47. Martino, J. Metabolic Alterations Induced by High Maternal BMI and Gestational Diabetes in Maternal, Placental and Neonatal Outcomes. Ph.D. Thesis, The University of Nottingham, Nottingham, UK, 2013.
48. Symonds, M.E.; Bloor, I.; Ojha, S.; Budge, H. The placenta, maternal diet and adipose tissue development in the newborn. *Ann. Nutr. Metab.* **2017**, *70*, 232–235. [CrossRef] [PubMed]

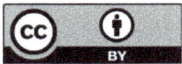

Article

Selenium Intake in Iodine-Deficient Pregnant and Breastfeeding Women in New Zealand

Ying Jin [1], Jane Coad [2], Janet L Weber [2], Jasmine S Thomson [2] and Louise Brough [2,*]

[1] School of Health Sciences, College of Health, Massey University, Palmerston North 4442, New Zealand;
    y.jin@massey.ac.nz
[2] School of Food and Advanced Technology, College of Sciences, Massey University, Palmerston North 4442,
    New Zealand; j.coad@massey.ac.nz (J.C.); j.l.weber@massey.ac.nz (J.L.W.); j.a.thomson@massey.ac.nz (J.S.T.)
*   Correspondence: l.brough@massey.ac.nz; Tel.: +64-6-951-7575

Received: 30 November 2018; Accepted: 18 December 2018; Published: 1 January 2019

✅ check for updates

Abstract: Selenium plays a role in antioxidant status and, together with iodine, in thyroid function. Iodine deficiency exists in New Zealand during pregnancy and lactation, and selenium deficiency may further affect thyroid function. This study investigated selenium intakes of pregnant and lactating women, in Palmerston North, in the North Island of New Zealand. Dietary intake was estimated using three repeated 24-h dietary recalls. Dietary intake in pregnancy was also estimated from 24-h urinary excretion of selenium. Selenium concentrations were determined in urine and breastmilk using inductively-coupled plasma mass spectrometry. Median selenium intakes based on dietary data were 51 (39, 65) μg/day in pregnancy and 51 (36, 80) μg/day in lactation, with 61% and 68% below estimated average requirement (EAR). Median daily selenium intake in pregnancy based on urinary excretion was 49 (40, 60) μg/day, with 59% below EAR. Median selenium concentration in breastmilk was 11 (10, 13) μg/L and estimated median selenium intake for infants was 9 (8, 10) μg/day, with 91% below the Adequate Intake of 12 μg/day. These pregnant and breastfeeding women were at risk of dietary selenium inadequacy. Further research is required to assess selenium status in relation to thyroid function and health in this group.

Keywords: selenium; pregnancy; lactation; breastfeeding; infants

---

1. Introduction

The intake of selenium worldwide ranges from 7 to 4990 μg/day, and varies greatly from deficient to toxic intakes [1]. New Zealand soils contain low levels of selenium, leading to low levels in the food supply [2]. The most recent New Zealand Total Diet Survey suggested dietary selenium intake was inadequate throughout the New Zealand population, putting them at risk of deficiency [3]. Recent New Zealand studies have shown low selenium intakes in women of childbearing age and older women based on urinary selenium excretion [4,5].

Selenium is essential in human health to produce selenoproteins, which have antioxidant and anti-inflammatory roles, and also for production of thyroid hormones [6]. Selenoproteins (iodothyronine deiodinases) are required for generating the active thyroid hormone T_3 (triiodothyronine) from the inactive T_4 (thyroxine) form [7]. Selenium is also an essential cofactor for glutathione peroxidase, a potent antioxidant, which protects thyroid cells from damage due to any excessive hydrogen peroxide generated from the synthesis of thyroid hormones [8].

Selenium has been suggested to play an important role in normal brain development, although the mechanism is not clear. Two recent large cohort studies from Poland and Spain found selenium status in first trimester was adversely associated with neuropsychological development assessed at 1 year and 2 years of age by the Bayley Scales of infants and Toddler development [9], and 5 years of age by the McCarthy Scales for Children's Abilities (MSCA) [10]. Varsi et al. (2017) investigated the effect of maternal selenium status on neurodevelopment of infants and reported that low serum selenium concentration in pregnancy was negatively associated with infant psychomotor score at 6 months of age [11].

The interaction between selenium and iodine in thyroid hormone synthesis is of particular concern in New Zealand due to dietary insufficiency of both selenium and iodine. Iodine deficiency has historically been a health problem in New Zealand [12] and the mandatory fortification of all bread (except organic) with iodised salt was introduced in September 2009 [13]. Since mandatory fortification, the majority of adults [14] and school-aged children [15] in New Zealand have adequate iodine intakes. Despite an iodine supplement being recommended and available to all pregnant and lactating women in New Zealand, this population group still has insufficient intakes and low status [16]. Selenium deficiency could potentially exacerbate the consequences of mild iodine deficiency among this vulnerable group [12].

During pregnancy and lactation, there are increased selenium requirements for the growing foetus and newborn [3]. Low maternal serum selenium concentrations are associated with adverse pregnancy outcomes such as pre-eclampsia [17], other types of pregnancy-induced hypertension [18] and preterm birth [19]. Human milk is critical for an exclusively breastfed infant's optimal selenium status. A study in the South Island of New Zealand (1998–1999) showed postpartum women and breastfed infants had low plasma selenium, suggesting suboptimal status [20]. Since then, no data about selenium intakes have been collected for this population. Given changes in dietary habits, food product availability and agricultural practices, continual monitoring of selenium intake in this vulnerable population is essential.

This study aimed to assess current maternal selenium intake during pregnancy and lactation, and estimate infant selenium intake in a sample of women in Palmerston North, North Island, New Zealand.

2. Materials and Methods

2.1. Study Population

Pregnant and breastfeeding women were recruited from January to July 2009 and January to September 2011 via local health professionals who work closely with pregnant and breastfeeding women, as described previously [16]. Volunteers were aged 16 years and older, in their third trimester of pregnancy (greater than 26 weeks of gestation), or at least 3 weeks postpartum and breastfeeding. Women who had medical complications during their pregnancy were excluded. In total, 59 pregnant and 68 lactating women were recruited and included in the study. Women had to actively volunteer for this study and no data were kept from women who did not meet the selection criteria.

Ethical approval was obtained from the Massey University Human Ethics Committee (Southern A 08/32 and 10/54). Written consent was obtained from all participants.

2.2. Dietary Data Collection

A 24-h dietary recall was conducted based on the US Department of Agriculture Automated Multiple-Pass Method, but excluded the Forgotten Foods List [21]. A photographic food atlas was provided to estimate portion sizes [22]. Participants were also asked to include any dietary supplements taken, including the brand name and the amount. Two subsequent recalls were collected via telephone interviews over the following two weeks, ensuring a weekend day was included; food portion sizes were estimated using household measures. Previous research has found no difference in energy intakes when comparing 24-h dietary recalls collected in person versus via the telephone [23]. Dietary data were analysed using Foodworks 2009 (Xyris Software, Brisbane, Australia) based on the New Zealand food database. Dietary supplements used by participants were included in dietary data analysis. Only 4 of the 59 pregnant and 6 of the 68 lactating women were taking selenium-containing supplements.

The estimated average requirement (EAR) cut-point method can be used to assess population nutrient intake providing nutrient requirements are normally distributed (e.g., selenium); the percentage below the EAR approximates the proportion that is at risk of dietary inadequacy [24]. For a population to have a very low prevalence of inadequate dietary intakes, the mean/median intake should be above the recommended daily intake (RDI) [24]. Current intakes based on diet and urine data were compared to Australian and New Zealand recommendations; the Estimated Average Requirement (EAR) and Recommended Dietary Intake (RDI) for selenium for pregnant women are 55 and 65 μg/day, and for lactating women are 65 and 75 μg/day, respectively [3].

2.3. Sample Collection and Selenium Analysis of Urine and Breastmilk

All participants were asked to collect a 24-h urine sample and provided with an insulated box containing two polythene bottles for urine storage and frozen silica pads to keep the sample cool. Lactating women were also requested to provide a breastmilk sample (around 30 mL) and provided with a breast pump if required; timing of collection of breastmilk samples was not standardized, since no significant differences have been found in selenium concentrations between hind-milk and fore-milk [25]. The concentration of selenium in breastmilk varies most significantly during the first 21 days from the transition from colostrum to mature milk [25], thus breastmilk samples were collected after 3 weeks postpartum. All samples were brought immediately to the Human Nutrition Research Unit for processing after collection. The total volume of urine collected over 24 h was measured for each participant. Samples were stored without preservative at −20 °C, prior to analysis. Urine samples were defined as inaccurate if urine volume was below 1 L and urinary creatinine below 5 mmol/day, or extreme outliers of creatinine (>3 Standard Deviation) [26]. However, no study samples were classified accordingly.

Selenium concentrations of urine and breastmilk samples were determined by Hill Laboratories, Hamilton, New Zealand, using inductively-coupled plasma mass spectrometry [27]. Quality Control procedures included analysis of blanks, analytical repeats and spiked samples in order to ensure accuracy and precision. Calibration standards and checks were undertaken on every run with the limit of detection at 0.002 mg/kg. Dietary selenium intake was estimated for pregnant women, based on a urinary excretion of 55% of selenium intake [28]. However, it was not possible to estimate dietary selenium intake for lactating women via urine, as we were unable to determine the daily loss of selenium from breastmilk. Creatinine was measured using the Jaffe Method Flexor E (Vital Scientific NV, 6956 AV Spankeren/Dieren, Rheden, Gelderland, The Netherlands) at Massey University Nutrition Laboratory.

2.4. Statistical Analysis

Data were analysed using IBM SPSS (Statistics Package for the Social Sciences, IBM, Armonk, NY, USA) version 20. Data were tested for normality using Shapiro-Wilk's test. Non-parametric data were expressed as median (Quartile 1, 3 (Q1, Q3); based on weighted average) and parametric data expressed as mean (±standard deviation; SD). Bivariate correlations were tested using the nonparametric Spearman's rho correlation coefficient. Scatter plots were generated for suspected bivariate correlations and visually inspected for verification. Fisher's exact test was used to detect associations between dietary and biological methods in assessing dietary intake.

3. Results

Fifty-nine pregnant and 68 lactating women were recruited. The mean age was 31.6 ± 5.7 and 31.3 ± 5.0 years for pregnant and breastfeeding women, respectively (Table 1). The ethnicities of participants were Caucasian (80%, 81%), Maori (12%, 9%), Asian (5%, 2%) and other (3%, 8%). Participants were predominantly educated at tertiary level (86% pregnant and 68% breastfeeding), with approximately half being pregnant with or breastfeeding their first infant.

Nutrients **2019**, *11*, 69

Table 1. Description of pregnant and breastfeeding participants.

n (%)	Pregnant	Breastfeeding
	n = 59	n = 68
Age, years (Mean ± SD)	31.6 ± 5.7	31.3 ± 5.0
Tertiary Education	51 (86)	46 (68)
Ethnicity (Caucasian)	47 (80)	56 (81)
Ethnicity (Maori)	7 (12)	6 (9)
Ethnicity (Asian)	3 (5)	1 (2)
Ethnicity (Other)	2 (3)	5 (7)
Nulliparous	31 (53)	-
First time lactation	-	36 (53)
Gestational age, days (Median (Q1, Q3))	207 (191, 247)	
Age of infants, days (Mean ± SD)		113.4 ± 96.9

Median urinary selenium for pregnant women was 14.1 (9.1, 18.2) µg/L (Table 2) and median selenium intake based on urinary excretion was 49 (40, 60) µg/day (Table 3), below both the RDI (65 µg/day) and EAR (55 µg/day), with 59% below the EAR. Median selenium intake based on dietary assessment among pregnant women was 51 (39, 65) µg/day, below both the RDI and EAR, with 61% below the EAR (Table 3). Urinary and dietary data both suggest inadequate selenium intakes among pregnant participants.

Table 2. Selenium and creatinine in 24-h urine samples from pregnant and breastfeeding women and selenium in breastmilk from breastfeeding women.

Median (Q1, Q3)	Pregnant	Breastfeeding
Numbers of participants (n)	59	68
Urine volume (L)	2.2 (1.5, 3.0)	1.8 (1.2, 2.5)
Urinary selenium concentration µg/L	14.1 (9.1, 18.2)	12.1 (7.8, 19.9)
Measured 24-h urinary selenium µg/day	27.1 (22.0, 32.9)	21.2 (14.5, 29.9)
Urinary creatinine g/L	0.5 (0.4, 0.7)	0.7 (0.5, 1.1)
Urinary creatinine g/day	1.2 (1.0, 1.5)	1.3 (1.2, 1.4)
Selenium: creatinine µg/g	22.8 (17.7, 28.7)	16.5 (12.3, 23.8)
Selenium in breastmilk µg/L	-	11.3 (10.0, 13.3) [a]

[a] n = 64 for breastmilk samples.

Table 3. Estimated selenium intake in pregnant and breastfeeding women, infants and comparison to recommendations.

Selenium Intake	Pregnant	Breastfeeding	Infant
	(n = 59)	(n = 68)	(n = 64)
Estimated selenium intake; median (Q1, Q3)			
Based on 24-h urine, µg/day	49 (40, 60)		
Based on 24-h dietary recalls, µg/day	51 (39, 65)	51 (36, 80)	-
[a] Below EAR (n, %)			
Based on 24-h urine	35 (59)		
Based on 24-h dietary recalls	36 (61)	45 (68)	-
Estimated selenium intake; median (Q1, Q3)			
Based on 750 mL breastmilk per day	-	-	9 (8, 10)
Below (10 µg/day) (n, %)	-	-	45 (70)
Below (12 µg/day) (n, %)	-	-	58 (91)

[a] EAR = estimated average requirement, 55 µg/day for pregnant women and 65 µg/day for breastfeeding women.

Based on dietary assessment, the median selenium intake for breastfeeding women was 51 (36, 80) µg/day (Table 3), also below both the EAR (65 µg/day) and RDI (75 µg/day), with 68%

below the EAR. Median selenium concentration in breastmilk (n = 64) was 11 (10, 13) µg/L (Table 2). Using an estimated daily breastmilk intake of 750 mL [29], the median estimated selenium intake for infants was 9 (8, 10) µg/day; 70% (45/64) were below the daily minimum of 10 µg/day suggested by Levander [30], and 91% (58/64) below the Adequate Intake of 12 µg/day [31].

For breastfeeding women, selenium concentration in breastmilk was weakly positively correlated with 24-h selenium excretion in urine as µg/day (p = 0.269, r = 0.032, see Table A2). Pregnant participants' dietary selenium intake based on dietary assessment was not associated with selenium excretion as either µg/L (p = 0.053, r = 0.692) or µg/day (p = 0.230, r = 0.079; see Table A1). However, the classifications of intakes as either above or below the EAR were associated for the two methods of assessing dietary intake (p = 0.016, Fisher's exact test).

4. Discussion

This study found 59–61% of pregnant and 68% breastfeeding participants had estimated selenium intakes below the EAR, suggesting this vulnerable group is at risk of an inadequate selenium intake. This supports the latest New Zealand Adult Nutrition Survey 2008/2009, which estimated that 44–72% of women aged 19–50 years had inadequate selenium intakes [32]. Previous research shows that low selenium status is associated with an increased risk of thyroid enlargement, which may indicate compromised thyroid function [33]. Iodine deficiency has previously been reported in both pregnant and breastfeeding women in New Zealand in the same cohort investigated in this study [16], and selenium deficiency could further compromise thyroid function.

In the present study, dietary intake was assessed by three 24-h dietary recalls, due to its low participant burden and good compliance. Under- or over-reporting is a concern for dietary assessment. As energy expenditure was not recorded, we were unable to determine if participants had misreported dietary intake. A large daily variation of selenium intake was reported in an earlier study of American pregnant and postpartum women using duplicate-plate food and drink composites and dietary recalls [34]. Single 24-h recalls do not take into account day-to-day variation, therefore repeated 24-h dietary recalls are frequently used to estimate usual intake [35].

In the current study, 24-h urinary selenium excretion was used to estimate selenium intake. It is estimated that 50–60% of dietary selenium is excreted in urine [28], and selenium intake determined in this manner is suggested to be more accurate than dietary assessment data [36]. However, collecting 24-h urine samples requires motivated participants and is not practical for all populations or large studies. Urinary selenium has been shown to be a valid method to assess recent selenium intake in populations that live in selenium-deficient areas [36,37]. Research has shown that serum selenium and glomerular filtration rate increase in pregnancy, and studies have shown an increase in selenium in urine during pregnancy [38]. Thus, the selenium excretion of 55% could be overestimated, so actual selenium intakes could be even lower than estimated values. A previous New Zealand study found selenium intake determined from a Food Frequency Questionnaire was associated with 24-h urine excretion in pregnant women [38]. Although the current study found no such association in pregnant women, the classification of intakes as either above or below the EAR was associated for the two methods of assessing dietary intake.

Median intake of selenium for pregnant women in the current study was 51 µg/day based on dietary intake and 49 µg/day based on urine excretion. In previous studies of New Zealand pregnant women, Watson and McDonald found median intakes ranging between 33.5 µg/day excluding dietary supplements to 67 mcg/day including dietary supplements [39], however, these data were based on dietary assessment with no verification using biomarkers. The median selenium intake of 51 µg/day for breastfeeding women was higher than previously reported (46 µg/day) in the 1998–1999 study of lactating mothers from the South Island of New Zealand [20]. This was not unexpected, as selenium intake is typically lower in the South Island of New Zealand, where bread is made from local wheat, compared to the North Island, where bread is manufactured from wheat imported from Australia, which has higher levels of soil selenium [12]. It could also be due to changes occurring in diet in the last 20 years. Even though selenium intake is higher among breastfeeding women in the current study than previously reported, many current intakes are still below the EAR, thus suggesting a risk of dietary inadequacy.

Breastmilk selenium concentration is associated with maternal selenium intake and/or status. Selenium is generally higher in colostrum (26 µg/L), and then decreases to nadir levels in mature milk (1–3 months, 15 µg/L) [30]. Median selenium breastmilk concentrations (11.3 µg/L) in the present study were similar to those reported in the South Island in 1992 (13.4 µg/L) [40] and also a recent study in the North Island (14 µg/L) [41]. Adequate selenium concentrations in breastmilk have been observed to maintain optimum selenium status in both preterm and term infants [25]. For exclusively breastfed infants, breastmilk is the only source of selenium; in the current study, 70% of infants would not have achieved the 10 µg/day suggested as adequate by extrapolation from adults [30] and 91% did not achieve the Adequate Intake of 12 µg/day [18]. This suggests infants in the present study are at risk of selenium deficiency.

The inadequate selenium intakes in this vulnerable population are of concern. Studies in rats have previously shown that in utero selenium deficiency can impair neonatal lung development [42]. Maternal selenium status in French women was negatively associated with risk of wheezing in children aged 1–3 years; this could potentially lead to asthma later in life [43]. Low selenium status in childhood in New Zealand has also been associated with increased risk of wheeze [44], for which New Zealand has a high incidence [45]. Low maternal selenium status in Norwegian women has been associated with an increased risk of neonatal infections in the first 6 weeks of life and lower psychomotor score at 6 months [11]. Adequate dietary intake of selenium has been suggested to be beneficial in improving mental outlook among the general population [46]. Lower dietary selenium intake has also been associated with an increased risk of de novo major depressive disorder among women [47]. Selenium supplementation during early pregnancy has been found to reduce postnatal depression [48], which has a 7.8% to 16% prevalence in New Zealand [49].

Determining selenium concentrations in blood (whole, plasma or erythrocyte), plasma selenium protein P or GPx activity in blood (whole, plasma or platelet) are considered more reliable markers of selenium status [50,51]. However, urinary selenium excretion is associated with both plasma selenium and dietary intake in populations with low selenium intake [12]. A limitation of the current study is not measuring selenium or GPx activity in blood, however, determining daily urinary selenium excretion serves as a proxy measure for selenium intake and indicates the need for further research.

This study included a small sample of pregnant and breastfeeding women who were predominantly well educated and more likely to be affluent, thus the sample is not representative of the New Zealand population. However, women who volunteer for health studies tend to be interested in health and motivated towards a healthy lifestyle, thus it is of concern that these women are at risk of selenium deficiency. Further, we would not expect such women to have a poorer health status than less affluent women.

Additionally, supplement intakes could contribute to participants' dietary selenium intake; however, only a small proportion of participants consumed selenium-containing supplements. Thus, we were not able to meaningfully investigate the potential impact of supplement intake on other measures.

5. Conclusions

This current research suggests dietary selenium intake is a concern for pregnant and breastfeeding women and their infants in New Zealand. Further research is required to assess selenium status among these groups by measuring biomarkers such as plasma selenium or GPx activity in blood selenium. Further investigations should also include all socio-economic groups. It is essential that we assess whether suboptimal intake of selenium adversely affects thyroid function in this already iodine-deficient population. As selenium is a nutrient with numerous roles, it is also necessary to investigate any effects of low intake on other health outcomes potentially related to selenium in the perinatal period, such as postnatal depression and infant neurodevelopment.

Author Contributions: Conceptualization: Y.J., J.C., J.C., J.L.W., J.S.T. and L.B.; Formal analysis: Y.J. and L.B.; Funding acquisition: L.B.; Investigation: Y.J.; Supervision: J.C. and L.B.; Writing—original draft: Y.J.; Writing—review and editing: J.C., J.L.W., J.S.T. and L.B.

Acknowledgments: This study was funded by Palmerston North Medical Research Foundation and Massey University Research Fund.

Conflicts of Interest: The authors declare no conflict of interest. The funding sponsors had no role in the design of the study; in the collection, analyses, or interpretation of data; in the writing of the manuscript, and in the decision to publish the results.

Appendix A

Table A1. Correlation matrix for selenium and creatinine in 24-h urine samples in pregnant women using Spearman's rho.

n = 59		Urine	Urine Selenium	Estimated Selenium Intake (Urine)	Urine Creatinine	Urine Creatinine	Selenium: Creatinine Ratio	Estimated Selenium Intake (Dietary Data)
		Volume L	µg/L	µg/day	g/L	g/day	µg/g	µg/day
Urine Selenium µg/L	r	−0.719						
	p	0.000						
Estimated Selenium Intake (Urine) µg/day	r	ns	0.485					
	p		0.000					
Urine Creatinine g/L	r	−0.863	0.760	ns				
	p	0.000	0.000					
Urine Creatinine g/day	r	ns	ns	0.380	0.259			
	p			0.003	0.047			
Selenium Creatinine Ratio µg/g	r	ns	0.466	0.804	ns	ns		
	p		0.000	0.000				
Estimated Selenium Intake (Dietary Data) µg/day	r	ns	ns	0.230	ns	ns	ns	
	p			0.079 (ns)				
Total Energy Intake kJ	r	ns	ns	ns	ns	ns	ns	0.263
	p							0.044

ns = not statistically significant.

Table A2. Correlation matrix for selenium and creatinine in 24-h urine samples in breastfeeding women using Spearman's rho.

n = 68		Urine Volume L	Urine Selenium µg/L	Urine Selenium µg/day	Urine Creatinine g/L	Urine Creatinine g/day	Selenium: Creatinine Ratio µg/g	Milk Selenium µg/L	Dietary Selenium µg/day
Urine Selenium µg/L	r	−0.631							
	p	0.000							
Urine Selenium µg/day	r	ns	0.642						
	p		0.000						
Urine Creatinine g/L	r	−0.871	0.657	ns					
	p	0.000	0.000						
Urine Creatinine g/day	r	ns	ns	ns	ns				
	p								
Selenium Creatinine Ratio µg/g	r	ns	0.580	0.879	ns	ns			
	p		0.000	0.000					
Milk Selenium µg/day	r	ns	ns	0.269	ns	ns	0.280	ns	
	p			0.000			0.025		
Dietary Selenium µg/day	r	ns	ns	ns	−0.357	ns	ns	ns	
	p				0.003				
Total Energy Intake	r	0.247	ns	ns	ns	ns	ns	ns	0.405
	p	0.043							0.001

References

1. Rayman, M.P. The Importance of Selenium to Human Health. *Lancet* **2000**, *356*, 233–241. [CrossRef]
2. Stewart, R.D.; Griffiths, N.M.; Thomson, C.D.; Robinson, M.F. Quantitative selenium metabolism in normal New Zealand women. *Br. J. Nutr.* **1978**, *40*, 45–54. [CrossRef] [PubMed]
3. National Health and Medicine Council, New Zealand Ministry of Health. *Nutrient Reference Values for Australia and New Zealand Including Recommended Dietary Intake*; National Health and Medicine Council, New Zealand Ministry of Health: Canberra, Australia, 2006.
4. Shukri, N.H.; Coad, J.; Weber, J.; Jin, Y.; Brough, L. Iodine and Selenium Intake in a Sample of Women of Childbearing Age in Palmerston North, New Zealand after Mandatory Fortification of Bread with Iodised Salt. *Food Nutr. Sci.* **2014**, *2014*, 382–389. [CrossRef]
5. Brough, L.; Gunn, C.A.; Weber, J.L.; Coad, J.; Jin, Y.; Thomson, J.S.; Mauze, M.; Kruger, M.C. Iodine and Selenium Intakes of Postmenopausal Women in New Zealand. *Nutrients* **2017**, *9*, 254. [CrossRef] [PubMed]
6. Rayman, M.P. Selenium and human health. *Lancet* **2012**, *379*, 1256–1268. [CrossRef]
7. Schomburg, L.; Köhrle, J. On the importance of selenium and iodine metabolism for thyroid hormone biosynthesis and human health. *Mol. Nutr. Food Res.* **2008**, *52*, 1235–1246. [CrossRef] [PubMed]
8. Zimmermann, M.B.; Köhrle, J. The impact of iron and selenium deficiencies on iodine and thyroid metabolism: Biochemistry and relevance to public health. *Thyroid* **2002**, *12*, 867–878. [CrossRef]
9. Polanska, K.; Krol, A.; Sobala, W.; Gromadzinska, J.; Brodzka, R.; Calamandrei, G.; Chiarotti, F.; Wasowicz, W.; Hanke, W. Selenium status during pregancy and child psychomotor development—Polish Mother and Child Cohort study. *Padiatr. Res.* **2016**, *79*, 863–869. [CrossRef]
10. Amorós, R.; Murcia, M.; González, L.; Rebagliato, M.; Iñiguez, C.; Lopez-Espinosa, M.J.; Vioque, J.; Broberg, K.; Ballester, F.; Llop, S. Maternal selenium status and neuropychological development in Spanish preschool children. *Environ. Res.* **2018**, *166*, 215–222. [CrossRef]
11. Varsi, K.; Bolann, B.; Torsvik, I.; Constanse, T.; Eik, R.; Høl, P.J. Impact of Maternal Selenium Status on Infant Outcome during the First 6 Months of Life. *Nutrients* **2017**, *9*, 486. [CrossRef]
12. Thomson, C.D. Selenium and iodine intakes and status in New Zealand and Australia. *Br. J. Nutr.* **2004**, *91*, 661–672. [CrossRef] [PubMed]
13. Food Standards Australia New Zealand. *Australia New Zealand Food Standards Code, Standard 2.1.1. Cereals and Cereal Products*; Food Standards Australia New Zealand: Barton, Australia, 2015.
14. Edmonds, J.; McLean, R.; Williams, S.; Skeaff, S. Urinary iodine concentration of New Zealand adults improves with mandatory fortification of bread with iodised salt but not to predicted levels. *Eur. J. Nutr.* **2016**, *55*, 1201–1212. [CrossRef] [PubMed]
15. Jones, E.; McLean, R.; Davies, B.; Hawkins, R.; Meiklejohn, E.; Ma, Z.F.; Skeaff, S. Adequate Iodine Status in New Zealand School Children Post-Fortification of Bread with Iodised Salt. *Nutrients* **2016**, *8*, 298. [CrossRef] [PubMed]
16. Brough, L.; Jin, Y.; Shukri, N.H.; Wharemate, Z.R.; Weber, J.L.; Coad, J. Iodine intake and status during pregnancy and lactation before and after government initiatives to improve iodine status, in Palmerston North, New Zealand: A pilot study. *Matern. Child Nutr.* **2015**, *11*, 646–655. [CrossRef] [PubMed]
17. Mistry, H.D.; Wilson, V.; Ramsay, M.M.; Symonds, M.E.; Pipkin, F.B. Reduced selenium concentrations and glutathione peroxidase activity in preeclamptic pregnancies. *Hypertension* **2008**, *52*, 881–888. [CrossRef] [PubMed]
18. Rayman, M.P.; Bath, S.C.; Westaway, J.; Williams, P.; Mao, J.; Vanderlelie, J.J.; Perkins, A.V.; Redman, C.W. Selenium status in UK pregnant women and its relationship with hypertensive conditions of pregnancy. *Br. J. Nutr.* **2015**, *113*, 249–258. [CrossRef] [PubMed]
19. Rayman, M.; Wijnen, H.; Vader, H.; Kooistra, L.; Pop, V. Maternal selenium status during early gestation and risk for preterm birth. *CMAJ* **2011**, *183*, 549–555. [CrossRef]
20. McLachlan, S.K.; Thomson, C.D.; Ferguson, E.L.; McKenzie, J.E. Dietary and biochemical selenium status of urban 6- to 24-month-old South Island New Zealand children and their postpartum mothers. *J. Nutr.* **2004**, *134*, 3290–3295. [CrossRef]
21. Moshfegh, A.J.; Rhodes, D.G.; Baer, D.J.; Murayi, T.; Clemens, J.C.; Rumpler, W.V.; Paul, D.R.; Sebastian, R.S.; Kuczynski, K.J.; Ingwersen, L.A.; et al. The US Department of Agriculture Automated Multiple-Pass Method reduces bias in the collection of energy intakes. *Am. J. Clin. Nutr.* **2008**, *88*, 324–332. [CrossRef]

22. Nelson, N.; Atkinson, M.; Meyer, J. *Food Portion Size: A User's Guide to the Photographic Atlas*; Ministry of Agriculture Fisheries and Food: London, UK, 1997.

23. Tran, K.M.; Johnson, R.K.; Soultanakis, R.P.; Matthews, D.E. In-person vs telephone-administristered multiple-pas 24-hour recalls in women: Validation with doubly labeled water. *J. Am. Diet. Assoc.* **2000**, *100*, 777–780. [CrossRef]

24. Institute of Medicine. *Dietary Reference Intakes: Applications in Dietary Assessment*; National Academy Press: Washington, DC, USA, 2000.

25. Dorea, J.G. Selenium and breast-feeding. *Br. J. Nutr.* **2002**, *88*, 443–461. [CrossRef] [PubMed]

26. Huggins, C.E.; O'Reilly, S.; Brinkman, M.; Hodge, A.; Giles, G.G.; English, D.R.; Nowson, C.A. Relationship of urinary sodium and sodium-to-potassium ratio to blood pressure in older adults in Australia. *Med. J. Aust.* **2011**, *195*, 128–132. [PubMed]

27. Fecher, P.; Goldmann, I.; Nagengast, A. Determination of iodine in food samples by inductively coupled plasma mass spectrometry after alkaline extraction. *J. Anal. At. Spectrom.* **1998**, *13*, 977–982. [CrossRef]

28. Thomson, C.D. Assessment of requirements for selenium and adequacy of selenium status: A review. *Eur. J. Clin. Nutr.* **2004**, *58*, 391–402. [CrossRef] [PubMed]

29. Neville, C.; Seacat, J.; Casey, C. Studies in human lactation: During the onset of lactation milk volumes in lactating and full lactation. *Am. J. Clin. Nutr.* **1988**, *48*, 1375–1386. [CrossRef] [PubMed]

30. Levander, O.A. Upper limit of selenium in infant formulas. *J. Nutr.* **1989**, *119* (Suppl. 12), 1869–1872. [CrossRef] [PubMed]

31. Vannoort, R.; Thomson, B. *2009 New Zealand Total Diet Study: Agricultural Compound Residues, Selected Contaminant and Nutrient Elements*; Ministry for Primary Industries: Wellington, New Zealand, 2009.

32. New Zealand Ministry of Health. *A Focus on Nutrition: Key Findings of the 2008/09 New Zealand Adult Nutrition Survey*; New Zealand Ministry of Health: Wellington, New Zealand, 2011.

33. Rasmussen, L.B.; Schomburg, L.; Köhrle, J.; Pedersen, I.B.; Hollenbach, B.; Hög, A.; Ovesen, L.; Perrild, H.; Laurberg, P. Selenium status, thyroid volume, and multiple nodule formation in an area with mild iodine deficiency. *Eur. J. Endocrinol.* **2011**, *164*, 585–590. [CrossRef]

34. Levander, O.A.; Moser, P.B.; Morris, V.C. Dietary selenium intake and selenium concentrations of plasma, erythrocytes, and breast milk in pregnant and postpartum lactating and nonlactating women. *Am. J. Clin. Nutr.* **1987**, *46*, 694–698. [CrossRef]

35. Gibson, R.S. Measuring food consumption of individuals. In *Principles of Nutrition Assessment*, 2nd ed.; Gibson, R.S., Ed.; Oxford University Press: New York, NY, USA; Oxford, UK, 2005; pp. 41–64.

36. Thomson, C.D.; Smith, T.E.; Butler, K.A.; Packer, M.A. An evaluation of urinary measures of iodine and selenium status. *J. Trace Elem. Med. Biol.* **1996**, *10*, 214–222. [CrossRef]

37. Alaejos, M.S.; Romero, C.D. Urinary selenium concentrations. *Clin. Chem.* **1993**, *39*, 2040–2052.

38. Thomson, C.D.; Packer, M.A.; Butler, J.A.; Duffield, A.J.; O'Donaghue, K.L.; Whanger, P.D. Urinary selenium and iodine during pregnancy and lactation. *J. Trace Elem. Med. Biol.* **2001**, *14*, 210–217. [CrossRef]

39. Watson, P.E.; Mcdonald, B.W. Major Influences on Nutrient Intake in Pregnant New Zealand Women. *Matern. Child Nutr.* **2009**, *13*, 695–706. [CrossRef]

40. Dolamore, B.A.; Brown, J.; Darlow, B.A.; George, P.M.; Sluis, K.B.; Winterbourn, C.C. Selenium status of Christchurch infants and the effect of diet. *N. Z. Med. J.* **1992**, *105*, 139–142.

41. Butts, C.A.; Hedderley, D.I.; Herath, T.D.; Paturi, G.; Glyn-Jones, S.; Wiens, F.; Stahl, B.; Gopal, P. Human milk composition and dietary intakes of breastfeeding women of different ethnicity from the manawatu-wanganui region of New Zealand. *Nutrients* **2018**, *10*, 1231. [CrossRef] [PubMed]

42. Kim, H.Y.; Picciano, M.F.; Wallig, M.A.; Milner, J.A. The Role of Selenium Nutrition in the Development of Neonatal Rat Lung. *Pediatr. Res.* **1991**, *29*, 440–445. [CrossRef] [PubMed]

43. Baız, N.; Chastange, J.; Ibanez, G.; Annesi-Maesano, I. Prenatal exposure to selenium may protect against wheezing in children by the age of 3. *Imunity Inflamm. Dis.* **2017**, *5*, 37–44. [CrossRef] [PubMed]

44. Thomson, C.D.; Wickens, K.; Miller, J.; Ingham, T.; Lampshire, P.; Epton, M.J.; Town, G.I.; Pattemore, P.; Crane, J.; Year Six New Zealand Asthma and Allergy Cohort Study Group (NZAACS6). Selenium status and allergic disease in a cohort of New Zealand children. *Clin. Exp. Allergy* **2012**, *42*, 560–567. [CrossRef] [PubMed]

45. The International Study of Asthma and Allergies in Childhood (ISAAC) Steering Committee. Worldwide variation in prevalence of symptoms of asthma, allergic rhinoconjunctivitis, and atopic eczema: ISAAC. *Lancet* **1998**, *351*, 1225–1232. [CrossRef]

46. Benton, D. Selenium intake mood and other aspects of psychological funtioning. *Nutr. Neurosci.* **2002**, *5*, 363–374. [CrossRef] [PubMed]

47. Pasco, J.A.; Jacka, F.N.; Williams, L.J.; Evans-Cleverdon, M.; Brennan, S.L.; Kotowicz, M.A.; Nicholson, G.C.; Ball, M.J.; Berk, M. Dietary selenium and major depression: A nested case-control study. *Complement. Ther. Med.* **2012**, *20*, 119–123. [CrossRef]

48. Mokhber, N.; Namjoo, M.; Tara, F.; Boskabadi, H.; Rayman, M.P.; Ghayour-Mobarhan, M.; Sahebkar, A.; Majdi, M.R.; Tavallaie, S.; Azimi-Nezhad, M.; et al. Effect of supplementation with selenium on postpartum depression: A randomized double-blind placebo-controlled trial. *J. Matern. Fetal Neonatal Med.* **2011**, *24*, 104–108. [CrossRef] [PubMed]

49. Campbell, S.; Norris, S.; Standfield, L.; Suebwongpat, A. *Screening for Postnatal Depression with in the Well Child Tamariki Ora Framework*; Health Services Assessment Collaboration (HSAC): Christchurch, New Zealand, 2008.

50. Ashton, K.; Hooper, L.; Harvey, L.; Hurst, R.; Casgrain, A.; Fairweather-Tait, S. Methods of assessment of selenium status in humans: A systematic review. *Am. J. Clin. Nutr.* **2009**, *89*, 2070S–2084S. [CrossRef] [PubMed]

51. Longnecker, M.P.; Stram, D.O.; Taylor, P.R.; Levander, O.A.; Howe, M.; Veillon, C.; McAdam, P.A.; Patterson, K.Y.; Holden, J.M.; Morris, J.S.; et al. Use of selenium concentration in whole blood, serum, toenails, or urine as a surrogate measure of selenium intake. *Epidemiology* **1996**, *7*, 384–390. [CrossRef] [PubMed]

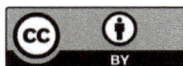

nutrients

MDPI

Article

Assessment of Dietary Intake and Nutrient Gaps, and Development of Food-Based Recommendations, among Pregnant and Lactating Women in Zinder, Niger: An Optifood Linear Programming Analysis

K. Ryan Wessells [1,*], **Rebecca R. Young** [1,†], **Elaine L. Ferguson** [2,†], **Césaire T. Ouédraogo** [1], **M. Thierno Faye** [3] **and Sonja Y. Hess** [1]

[1]   Program in International and Community Nutrition, Department of Nutrition, University of California, Davis, CA 95616, USA; rryoung@ucdavis.edu (R.R.Y.); ctouedraogo@ucdavis.edu (C.T.O.); syhess@ucdavis.edu (S.Y.H.)
[2]   Department of Population Health, London School of Hygiene and Tropical Medicine, London WC1E 7HT, UK; elaine.ferguson@lshtm.ac.uk
[3]   Helen Keller International, Niamey 0000, Niger; tfaye@hki.org
*   Correspondence: krwessells@ucdavis.edu; Tel.: +1-530-752-1992
†   The two authors contributed equally.

Received: 20 November 2018; Accepted: 20 December 2018; Published: 2 January 2019

check for
updates

Abstract: Pregnant and lactating women in rural Niger are at high risk for inadequate intakes of multiple micronutrients. Thus, 24 h dietary recalls were conducted and analyzed for dietary intakes in this population (n = 202). Using linear programming analyses, micronutrient gaps in women's diets were identified, food-based recommendations (FBR) to improve dietary micronutrient adequacy were developed, and various supplementation strategies were modelled. Energy intakes were below estimated requirements, and, for most micronutrients, >50% of women were at risk of inadequate intakes. Linear programming analyses indicated it would be difficult to select a diet that achieved recommended dietary allowances for all but three (vitamin B_6, iron and zinc) of 11 modeled micronutrients. Consumption of one additional meal per day, and adherence to the selected FBR (daily consumption of dark green leafy vegetables, fermented milk, millet, pulses, and vitamin A fortified oil), would result in a low percentage of women at risk of inadequate intakes for eight modeled micronutrients (vitamin A, riboflavin, thiamin, B_6, folate, iron, zinc, and calcium). Because the promotion of realistic FBRs likely will not ensure that a low percentage of women are at risk of inadequate intakes for all modeled micronutrients, multiple micronutrient supplementation or provision of nutrient-dense foods should be prioritized.

Keywords: linear programming; food-based recommendations; Optifood; micronutrient; deficiency; dietary intake; pregnant; lactation; women

---

1. Introduction

Maternal nutrition from the time of conception until two years post-partum, a period known as the first 1000 days, is critical for maternal and child health [1]. Undernutrition during pregnancy is a risk factor for maternal mortality and fetal growth restriction, which increases the risk of neonatal deaths and contributes to impaired post-natal linear growth and development [1]. Undernutrition during lactation adversely affects the concentrations of some macro- and micronutrients in breastmilk, which may negatively impact infant morbidity and mortality [2]. In low-income countries, it is particularly challenging for women to meet their macro- and micronutrient requirements during pregnancy and lactation [3]. In Niger, the lifetime risk of maternal death is 1 in 23 women and 11.4% of children die before reaching 5 years of age [4]. In a recent cross-sectional survey conducted among pregnant women in Zinder, Niger, 27% of pregnant women had inadequate gestational weight gain and 25% had low mid-upper arm circumference, indicative of undernutrition [5]. In addition, the prevalence of multiple micronutrient deficiencies was indicative of a severe public health problem. 45% of pregnant women were deficient in > 3 micronutrients (iron, zinc, vitamin A, folate, vitamin B_{12}), 79% were anemic, and less than 20% had adequate minimum dietary diversity [6]. Although information on the nutritional status of lactating women is limited, increased physiological requirements, frequent reproductive cycling and resource constraints make undernutrition likely. Overall, the Zinder region of Niger is considered a high risk livelihood zone, subject to severe food access constraints due in part to variable rainfall and frequent droughts, imbalanced agro-pastoralism, and high poverty levels. The 2011 National Survey on Living Conditions: Household and Agriculture in Niger (ECVMA) estimated that 47.7% of the population in the Zinder Region was living below the poverty line [7]. Chronic moderate and severe food insecurity affected 27.2% and 12.5% of the population in the Zinder region of Niger, respectively. During the lean season, these prevalences increased to 51.2% and 32.7%, respectively [7].

Evidence-based approaches to improve nutritional status among pregnant and lactating women include supplementation (e.g., iron and folic acid, multiple micronutrients, and balanced protein and energy supplementation), food fortification (e.g., mass fortification of cereals, oils, and condiments), and dietary counseling to promote the consumption of nutritionally dense foods [8–12]. Software tools for decision-making in nutrition programs have been developed to support advocacy and decision-making (e.g., Lives Saved Tool, LiST; Cost of the diet, COD), plan and optimize interventions (e.g., Intake Modeling, Assessment and Planning Program, IMAPP; Optifood), and optimize cost-benefits of combined interventions (e.g., MINIMOD) [13]. Optifood is based on the mathematical technique of linear programming, and was recently developed by the London School of Hygiene & Tropical Medicine, the World Health Organization (WHO) and USAID Food and Nutrition Technical Assistance Project (FANTA)/FHI 360. Optifood allows users to identify population-specific dietary nutrient gaps and develop food-based recommendations (FBR) centered on locally available and acceptable foods, accounting for existing dietary patterns and economic feasibility [14]. In addition, the approach can be used to evaluate the ability of existing and novel nutrient supplements and fortified foods to meet population-specific nutritional requirements [15–19], although it has, to date, primarily been used for infants and young children.

The primary objectives of the present study were to (1) assess dietary intake and nutritional adequacy among pregnant and lactating women in the Zinder region of Niger, (2) develop FBR for nutritional counseling accounting for current consumption patterns and the local availability of affordable nutrient-rich foods, and (3) identify any shortfalls requiring nutrient supplementation or fortification. The present study illustrates how the Optifood tool can be used to inform program and policy decisions regarding strategies to improve dietary adequacy among pregnant and lactating women in food insecure populations.

2. Materials and Methods

2.1. Study Design and Participants

The present assessment of dietary intake and daily nutrient intakes among pregnant and lactating women is a cross-sectional study embedded into the Niger Maternal Nutrition (NiMaNu) Project. The NiMaNu project was a program-based effectiveness trial in the Zinder region of Niger, designed to assist the Nigerien Ministry of Public Health in its efforts to improve the nutritional and health status of pregnant women through multiple strategies to increase antenatal care attendance and adherence to iron folic acid (IFA) supplementation. The overall NiMaNu programmatic intervention, study design and data collection methods have been reported in detail elsewhere [6,20,21]. Briefly, 18 governmental integrated health centers located in two districts (Zinder and Mirriah) of the Zinder Region of Niger were randomly assigned to time of enrollment in the NiMaNu project from March 2014–September 2015, and 2307 pregnant women in surrounding rural villages participated in the study. The present dietary intake assessment survey was implemented from May–October 2015, exclusive of the month of Ramadan and included women from nine villages within the catchment areas of three integrated health centers enrolled in the baseline NiMaNu survey during that time frame.

Pregnant and lactating women were identified using the random walk method [22] and were eligible to participate in the dietary intake assessment survey if they lived in the catchment area of the NiMaNu project, were in their second or third trimester of pregnancy or breastfeeding an infant or young child < 23 months of age from a singleton birth, were > 19 years of age, and provided written informed consent. Women were ineligible to participate if they were unable to provide consent due to impaired decision-making ability, or if they (or their breastfeeding child) had an illness warranting immediate hospital referral or a chronic or congenital illness interfering with dietary intake, as assessed via a structured questionnaire and the professional judgement of the fieldworkers and study coordinator (government certified midwives and medical doctor, respectively).

2.2. Ethical Considerations

The NiMaNu Project was approved by the National Ethical Committee in Niamey (Niger) (005/2013/CCNE; 007/MSP/CCNE/2015) and the Institutional Review Board of the University of California, Davis (USA) (447971). Consent materials were presented in both written and oral format, in the presence of a neutral witness. Informed consent was documented with a written signature or a fingerprint prior to enrollment in the study. The study was registered at www.clinicaltrials.gov as NCT01832688.

2.3. Data Collection

2.3.1. Socio-Demographic Characteristics and Anthropometry

Information on socio-economic and demographic characteristics of the woman and her household, pregnancy and health status, food security, and knowledge, attitudes and practices pertaining to antenatal care and nutrition were collected via structured interviews by trained female fieldworkers [6,20,21]. The survey on knowledge, attitudes and practices included questions of knowledge (e.g., benefits of IFA and recommended foods to consume during pregnancy and lactation), attitudes (e.g., perceived importance of IFA, reasons for compliance or non-compliance with IFA supplementation, and identification of foods they would like to consume in greater quantity during pregnancy and lactation), and practices (e.g., IFA consumption, changes to physical labor and dietary intakes during pregnancy and lactation). Household food insecurity was assessed using the Household Food Insecurity Access Scale (HFIAS) of the Food and Nutrition Technical Assistance/USAID [23]. Height, weight, mid-upper arm circumference (MUAC) and symphysis-fundal height were measured by trained and standardized anthropometrists. Lightly clothed women were weighed to 50 g precision (SECA 874, Seca, Hamburg, Germany) in duplicate. Women's height (SECA 213, Seca, Hamburg, Germany), MUAC (ShorrTape© Measuring Tape, Weigh and Measure, Olney, MD, USA) and, among pregnant women, symphysis-fundal height (ShorrTape© Measuring Tape, Weigh and Measure, Olney, MD, USA) were measured in duplicate to 0.1 cm precision. If the two measurements were >0.2 kg (weight) or >0.5 cm apart (height, MUAC, and symphysis-fundal height), a third measurement was taken and the mean of the two closest measurements was calculated. Undernutrition was defined as a MUAC < 23 cm among pregnant women or a BMI < 18.5 kg/m^2 among lactating women, respectively [24]. Gestational age was estimated as a weighted average of the following obtained information: reported last menstrual period, time elapsed since quickening, and two fundal height measurements taken approximately one month apart [20,25].

2.3.2. 24 h Recall Data Collection

Three trained fieldworkers administered interactive quantitative 24 h dietary recall interviews, following the multi-pass approach developed for use in rural populations in low-income countries with low rates of literacy; study-specific data collection forms are available on the Open Science Framework platform [20,26]. Single 24 h dietary recalls were conducted in all participants; duplicate 24 h dietary recalls were attempted in a sub-sample of women (20%). 24 h dietary recalls were proportionally collected on weekdays (Monday-Thursday) and weekends (Friday-Sunday). Participating women were visited twice in their homes, two days apart. At the first visit, two days prior to the scheduled 24 h dietary recall, the purpose of the dietary interview was explained and participants were given a pictorial chart of common foods and a cup and bowl to use for their individual portions on the following day, to stimulate recall and allow the women to more accurately estimate portion sizes. On the day of the 24 h dietary recall interview, fieldworkers used neutral probing questions to help participants recall all the foods and drinks they had consumed during the preceding 24 h period (pass one). After this list was obtained, fieldworkers probed for more specific descriptions of all items listed in the first pass (pass two; e.g., brand names, recipes, cooking methods, waste or non-consumed parts, etc.). In the third pass, portion sizes were estimated using an electronic scale (when commonly consumed foods and ingredients carried by fieldworkers or foods or ingredients still available in the household could be directly weighed), equivalent volumes of water or dry good consumed (e.g., dry beans, dry couscous), pre-calibrated local utensils, rulers, modeling clay or monetary value. Finally, the fourth pass was used to review the recall and ensure all items were included and recorded correctly. A dietary diversity score (minimum dietary diversity for women; MDD-W) was calculated using 24 h recall data [27]. In addition, for all food items reported on the 24 h recall, women were asked to report the number of times per week or month that each food was typically consumed. For recipes or mixed dishes that were prepared by the index woman, information was collected on the type and amounts of ingredients, cooking methods, the total amount of recipe prepared, and the proportion she consumed. For composite dishes not prepared by the respondent and for staple foods with little intra-recipe variability, general recipes were constructed by commissioning three local women to prepare each recipe, or by compiling individual recipes obtained from women enrolled in the dietary intake assessment survey. In all cases, weights of raw ingredients were averaged in proportion to the total amount of recipe prepared. For all measurements not directly expressed in grams of food consumed, conversion factors were collected by fieldworkers in triplicate (e.g., cost data from local markets, densities of specific foods to convert estimated volumes of water or grams of dry goods to grams of prepared food, etc.), and applied to collected data, such that all data were ultimately expressed in grams of food consumed. In addition, all data were expressed in total cost of food consumed, using fieldworker acquired cost data from local markets, market survey data (see below) and participant-reported data.

2.3.3. Market Survey

Market surveys were conducted over seventeen months in all primary markets of the NiMaNu study area. From May 2014–September 2015, these markets ($n = 10$) were surveyed a total of 55 times (Zinder regional market, $n = 26$; 9 local markets in the Mirriah district, $n = 29$). Information was collected on food availability and cost, using a structured questionnaire based on the National Survey of Household Budget and Consumption and pre-tested in local markets [28]. Data are expressed as cost per 100 g edible portion.

2.3.4. Food Composition Table

Food nutrient values were obtained from the Optifood internal reference food composition table, which contains nutrient composition data for approximately 2000 foods. Nutrient values for any food items not contained in the Optifood food composition table were compiled from the INFOODS

Regional Nutrient Database for West Africa, the WorldFood System International Mini-list, and the United States Department of Agriculture Nutrient Database for Standard Reference, Release 28 (USDA SR28) [29]. The phytate contents of foods, including adjustments for fermentation, were imputed from study-specific analyses of food samples, or where data were not available, from the IML or a database compiled by Wessells et al. [30]. Nutrient contents of raw foods in the food composition table, when consumed in the cooked state, were adjusted for nutrient losses during cooking using retention factors from the USDA [31]. Refuse factors, obtained from the aforementioned databases, were used to convert all reported food units to edible portions.

Nutritional information from commercially available foods was obtained to account for fortification. Vegetable oils were assumed to be fortified with retinyl palmitate at the minimum at-market concentration of 11 mg/kg, as established by the West African Economic and Monetary Union (UEMOA) standards [32]. Wheat flour was assumed to be fortified with iron (60 mg/kg) and folic acid (2.5 mg/kg) [33,34]. Maggi brand bouillon cubes were assumed to be fortified with iron at a concentration of 600 mg/kg (based on package labelling and independent laboratory analyses) [35]; for the present Optifood analyses, all bouillon cubes were considered fortified. The nutrient composition of supplements (IFA, UNICEF/WHO/UNU international multiple micronutrient preparation (UNIMMAP)) and supplemental food products (Supercereal (i.e., Corn Soy Blend Plus, CSB+), Small Quantity Lipid-Based Nutrient Supplements for pregnant and lactation women (SQ-LNS P&L), Plumpy'Mum) was obtained from manufacturers specifications; details are in Table S1.

2.3.5. Dietary Reference Intakes

The dietary reference intakes (DRI) of the Food and Nutrition Board (FNB) of the Institute of Medicine (IOM; National Academies, USA) were used for these analyses (Table S2) [36–40]. Estimated energy requirements (EER) were calculated using IOM predictive equations by physiological status (specific to 2nd or 3rd trimester among pregnant women, and 0–6 or >6 months post-partum among lactating women) and physical activity level (PAL; assumed active PAL 1.27). The acceptable macronutrient distribution ranges (AMDR) of dietary protein and fat were considered to be 10–35% and 20–35% of energy, respectively. Nutritional adequacy of eleven micronutrients was assessed (thiamin, riboflavin, niacin, folate, vitamins B_6, B_{12}, A and C and iron, zinc and calcium). The estimated average requirement (EAR) and recommended dietary allowance (RDA) for micronutrients were IOM DRI recommendations, with the exception of the iron bioavailability among lactating women and the calcium recommendations. Specifically, for lactating women, the fractional absorption of iron was assumed to be 10%, due to lower bioavailability which may be encountered in predominantly vegetarian diets with limited diversity; thus increasing recommendations above those set by the IOM, yet still in line with recommendations from the WHO [3,41]. DRI for pregnant women were not adjusted, due to increases in iron absorption during later pregnancy [42]. In addition, models were run using both the calcium recommendations set by the IOM, as well as those recommended by WHO/FAO for settings where animal source foods provide less than 20–40 g/day of protein [41].

2.4. Data Analyses

Data were entered using EpiData version 3.1 (EpiData Association, Odense, Denmark). Dietary data were prepared in RedCap and SAS System software for Windows release 9.4 (SAS Institute, Cary, NC, USA). Statistical analyses were completed with SAS System software for Windows release 9.4 (SAS Institute, Cary, NC, USA). Descriptive statistics were calculated for all variables. The distribution of usual micronutrient intakes and daily per capita reported cost of foods consumed was estimated using the National Cancer Institute (NCI) method to adjust for intra-individual variation in dietary intake; the EAR cut-point method was applied to estimate the prevalence of inadequate intake [43,44]. Differences in market availability and median prices of specific foods by season were analyzed using logistic regression with Firth's adjustment and the Kruskal Wallis test on ranked data, respectively.

Data are presented as mean ± SD for normally distributed variables (Shapiro-Wilk statistic, W > 0.97), and the median and IQR for non-normal values. The alpha value is 0.05.

2.5. Optifood Analyses

2.5.1. Preparation of Linear Programming Model Parameters

Summary statistics from the dietary intake assessment survey (24 h recalls), including a list of foods consumed, food serving sizes and food patterns, were used to define the linear programming model parameters. The list of foods consumed included those consumed by > 5% of each target group and nutrient-dense foods consumed by < 5% of the target group, but with the potential to be promoted for consumption. It excluded all non-nutritive foods. Food serving sizes were defined as the median serving size (grams/meal) among consumers of each food; for staple foods (i.e., "grains and grain products"), food serving sizes were defined as 75th percentile, to allow for adequate flexibility to modeled energy. The minimum and maximum number of meals per week that a food could be consumed was calculated using data from the food frequency questionnaires. Minimum frequency was defined as 0 servings/week; maximum frequency was defined as the 90th percentile of the food frequency distribution for each group (pregnant and lactating women), with a lower limit of 1 serving/week and an upper limit of 21 servings/week. Weekly food consumption patterns for specific food groups and food sub-groups were included in the model (minimum and 90th percentile) to ensure that the diets modeled conformed to the range of food patterns observed in the target group. Estimated median servings per week, for each food group, defined food group goals in one of the Module II goal programming models. If the median value was zero, then a value of 0.1 servings per week was entered to avoid division by zero. These aforementioned parameters were used to define the model constraint levels used in the linear programming models analyzed in the WHO Optifood Software (version 4.0.14.0).

2.5.2. Development of Modelled Diets

The Optifood linear programming software (Modules I to III) was used to check model parameters, identify problem nutrients in the current dietary patterns of the target groups and to develop and test population-specific FBR for pregnant and lactating women [14,45]. Nutritionally "best" diets for the target population were generated based on established constraints and goals to achieve or exceed nutrient requirements (one model) or to achieve median food group patterns and achieve or exceed nutrient requirements (another model). Results from these goal programming models identified nutritious food sources, problem nutrients and alternative food-based recommendations to test. Next, linear programming was used, in Module III, to compare alternative sets of these food-based recommendations for nutritional adequacy and cost. Independent models for each micronutrient simulated the minimized (worst-case scenario) and maximized (best-case scenario) values of the nutrient intake distribution and provided cost estimates for each scenario [45].

Two series of analyses were done using the Optifood software tool. In the first series of analyses, the model energy constraint was equal to the reported mean energy intake for each target group (1812 kcal/day and 2280 kcal/day for pregnant and lactating women, respectively), henceforth referred to as "reported diet" models. A second series of diets was then modeled, in which the model energy constraint was increased to approximate the provision of an "added meal" (~600 kcal) per day [46] among pregnant women (2415 kcal/day), or to match estimated energy requirements in lactating women (2622 kcal/day). Subsequently, series of linear programming models were run to test alternative intervention products (Table 1).

Table 1. Series of linear programming models developed, with alternative intervention products, using the Optifood software tool [1].

	Pregnant Women		Lactating Women	
	Model Energy Constraint [2] (kcal/day)	Modeled Intervention Product (per day)	Model Energy Constraint [2] (kcal/day)	Modeled Intervention Product (per day)
Reported diet	1811.9	—	2279.5	—
Reported diet + IFA (standard of care)	1811.9	1 IFA	—	—
Added meal diet	2414.8	—	2622.0	—
Added meal diet + IFA	2414.8	1 IFA	—	—
Added meal diet + UNIMMAP [3]	2418.8	1 UNIMMAP	2622.0	1 UNIMMAP
Added meal diet + Supercereal (CSB+) [3,4]	2418.8	1 serving of CSB+ (500 kcal)	2622.0	1 serving of CSB+ (500 kcal)
Added meal diet + SQ-LNS (P&L) [3]	2418.8	1 serving of SQ-LNS (118 kcal)	2622.0	1 serving of SQ-LNS (118 kcal)
Added meal diet + Plumpy'Mum [3]	2418.8	1 serving of Plumpy'Mum (515 kcal/day)	2622.0	1 serving of Plumpy'Mum (515 kcal/day)

[1] CSB+, corn soy blend plus; IFA, iron and folic acid supplement; SQ-LNS, small-quantity lipid-based nutrient supplement; P&L, pregnancy and lactation; —, not available. [2] Reported diet: model energy constraint equal to the reported mean energy intake for each target group; Added meal diet: model energy constraint increased above the report diet to approximate the provision of an "added meal" (~600 kcal) per day among pregnant women or to match estimated energy requirements in lactating women. [3] Series modeled with and without lower calcium recommendation (800 mg/day). [4] Series which included 1 serving of Supercereal per day also included 1 serving/day of vegetable oil (10.5–10.7 g) and 1–2 servings/day of sugar (6.3–8.5 g) per 100 g Supercereal serving, based on local food patterns and preparation recommendations.

"Problem" nutrients were defined as nutrients where the nutrient did not achieve 100% of the RDA in the maximized best-case scenario; these are nutrients that will likely remain inadequate in the population given the local food supply and food patterns, even if women were to follow the FBR. Dietary adequacy for each nutrient was defined as the worst-case scenario for that nutrient being > 65% of the RDA. A worst-case-scenario level ≥ 65% indicates, if women achieve the FBR, then a low percentage of the population would be at risk of inadequate intakes for that nutrient.

2.6. Sample Size

Sample size estimates for the collection of dietary data among pregnant and lactating women were based on sample sizes previously reported in the literature [15,47,48]. Based on this information, and including an attrition rate of 10%, it was planned to enroll 110 pregnant women concurrent to their participation in the NiMaNu study and 110 lactating women residing in the same catchment areas. Duplicate non-consecutive day 24 h recalls were attempted in 20% of enrolled women within seven days, in order to examine intra-individual variation in nutrient intake.

Due to study resources and logistics, it was not always possible to implement the NiMaNu study and dietary intake assessment survey simultaneously as planned. Thus, only 56 pregnant women participating in the NiMaNu study were also enrolled in the present dietary assessment survey; an additional 48 pregnant women were enrolled in the dietary intake assessment survey only or subsequent to their completion of the NiMaNu study. In all cases, recruitment procedures were the same and data for the dietary intake assessment survey were collected using identical protocols and fieldworkers. In addition, an oversampling of lactating women occurred in the first village due to a miscommunication with fieldworkers. Thus, a post-hoc random sample of enrolled lactating women from the first village who completed the 24 h dietary recall was included in the analyses (*n* = 20 of 41).

3. Results

A total sample of 202 participants (103 lactating women and 99 pregnant women) was retained for analyses (Figure 1). The survey was primarily conducted during the "lean" season, and the majority of women reported moderate or severe household food insecurity. Only 16% of women reported adequate dietary diversity and >20% of participants were undernourished (Table 2).

3.1. Usual Dietary Intakes

Energy intakes in pregnant and lactating women were substantially below EER, and pregnant women reported consuming significantly fewer calories than lactating women, despite similar EER ($p < 0.0001$) (Table 3). Among pregnant women, reported mean energy intake did not differ by trimester ($p = 0.548$). Median percent contribution of energy from carbohydrates (70%) was slightly above the upper limit of the AMDR, and those of protein and fat were at or slightly below the lower limit of the acceptable macronutrient distribution ranges (10% and 20%, respectively). Usual dietary intakes of vitamin A, thiamin, riboflavin, niacin, folate and vitamin C were inadequate among >50% of pregnant and lactating women; usual dietary calcium and vitamin B_{12} intakes were inadequate for all women. Median (IQR) daily per capita reported cost of foods consumed was 0.35 € (0.28, 0.45) and 0.39 € (0.30, 0.49) for pregnant and lactating women, respectively.

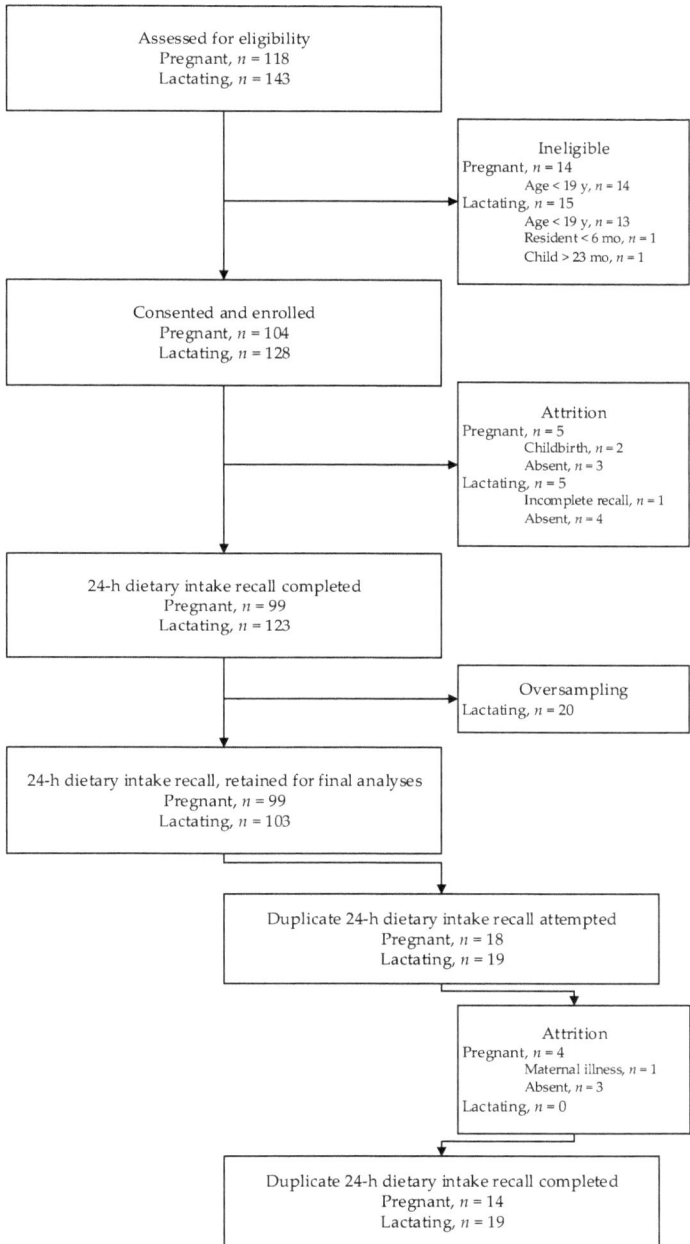

Figure 1. Flowchart of participant progression through the dietary intake assessment survey.

Table 2. Demographic characteristics of pregnant and lactating women and their households [1].

Variable	Pregnant	Lactating
Participants (*n*)	99	103
Age (years) [2]	27.8 ± 6.2	26.5 ± 6.4
Gravidity (*n*)	7.2 ± 3.3	—
Current pregnancy trimester		
Second, *n* (%)	59 (59.6)	—
Third, *n* (%)	40 (40.4)	—
Attended ANC in current pregnancy, *n* (%)	65 (65.7)	—
Age of breastfed child (months)	—	8.3 ± 5.6
Menses resumed, *n* (%)	—	26 (25.5)
Household food insecurity access scale (HFIAS), *n* (%)		
Food secure or mildly food insecure	48 (48.5)	43 (42.2)
Moderately food insecure	26 (26.3)	32 (31.3)
Severely food insecure	25 (25.3)	27 (26.5)
Daily per capita reported cost of foods consumed, € [3]	0.35 (0.28, 0.45)	0.39 (0.30, 0.49)
Daily per capita reported cost of foods below the national poverty line, % [4]	72.3	63.0
Received food rations in prior month, *n* (%)	6 (10.9) [5]	3 (2.9)
Adequate minimum dietary diversity – women (MDD-W), *n* (%)	16 (16.3)	15 (14.6)
Nutritional and health status		
Weight (kg)	56.4 ± 8.4	52.4 ± 9.0
BMI (kg/m²)	—	20.9 ± 3.2
Underweight (BMI <18.5 kg/m²)	—	22 (21.4)
Overweight (BMI >25 kg/m²)	—	9 (8.7)
Mid-upper arm circumference (cm)	25.1 ± 2.7	26.0 ± 2.9
MUAC <23 cm	20 (20.3)	3 (2.9)

[1] ANC, antenatal consultation; HFIAS, household food insecurity access scale; MDD-W, minimum dietary diversity –women; BMI, body mass index; MDD-W, minimum dietary diversity - women; MUAC, mid-upper arm circumference; —, not available. [2] Mean + SD, all such values. [3] Median (IQR); values calculated based on reported dietary intakes from 24 h dietary recalls using the National Cancer Institute (NCI) method to adjust for usual intake from [41,42]. [4] Cut-off values to define the national poverty line based on daily per capita food consumption expenditures, based on 2400 kcal food baskets and assuming an agro-pastoral system from [49]. [5] Data available for only *n* = 55 pregnant women; rations received by pregnant and lactating women included rice, millet, sorghum, beans, small-quantity lipid-based nutrient supplement and Supercereal.

Table 3. Median (IQR) usual daily dietary intakes of macro- and micronutrients from foods among pregnant and lactating women and prevalence of inadequate micronutrient intakes [1].

	Pregnant Women (n = 99)			Lactating Women (n = 103)		
	EAR [2]	Intake	Prevalence of Inadequacy (%)	EAR	Intake	Prevalence of Inadequacy (%)
Energy, kcal	2674.5	1759.7 (1475.5, 2101.3)		2622.2	2209.7 (1841.3, 2640.0)	
Vitamin A, μg RAE	550	536.1 [3] (378.4, 741.1)	52.1	900	504.9 (349.8, 701.6) [3]	88.8
Vitamin C, mg	70	25.9 (16.2, 39.7)	95.2	100	30.8 (19.3, 46.7)	97.9
Thiamin, mg	1.2	0.8 (0.7, 1.0)	89.3	1.2	1.0 (0.8, 1.2)	71.8
Riboflavin, mg	1.2	0.8 (0.6, 1.0)	91.8	1.3	0.9 (0.7, 1.2)	85.7
Niacin, mg	14	7.5 (6.4, 8.9)	98.4	13	9.1 (7.7, 10.8)	95.3
Vitamin B_6, mg	1.6	1.6 (1.3, 1.9)	52.1	1.7	2.0 (1.7, 2.5)	26.9
Folate, μg DFE	520	307.3 [3] (221.4, 414.7)	88.8	450	294.1 [3] (208.4, 398.8)	83.0
Vitamin B_{12}, μg	2.2	0.2 (0.1, 0.4)	100.0	2.4	0.3 (0.2, 0.5)	100.0
Iron, mg	22	22.6 [3] (17.5, 28.9)	46.7	11.7	30.1 [3] (23.6, 37.4)	1.0
Zinc, mg	9.5	11.0 (8.8, 13.7)	32.6	10.4	14.8 (11.9, 18.3)	14.3
Calcium, mg	800	330.3 (301.5, 361.5)	100.0	800	384.8 (351.0, 420.2)	100.0

[1] DFE, dietary folate equivalents; EAR, estimated average requirement; kcal, kilocalorie; RAE, retinol activity equivalent. [2] Estimated energy requirement (EER) = 354 − (6.91 × age [year]) + PA × [(9.36 × weight [kg]) + (726 × height [m])] + physiological group adjustment, where physical activity (PA) = 1.27 (active), and physiological group adjustments were as follows: 2nd trimester pregnancy = + 452; 3rd trimester pregnancy = + 330; 0–6 month postpartum = + 330; 7–23 months post-partum = + 400. [3] Assumes vitamin A fortification of cooking oil at 11 mg/kg from [31] and folic acid and iron fortification of wheat flour at 2.5 mg/kg and 60 mg/kg, respectively [32]. Does not include iron and folic acid supplements.

3.2. Optifood

3.2.1. Dietary Patterns and Linear Programming Model Parameters

Table S3 shows the foods commonly consumed by pregnant and lactating women, the median serving sizes among consumers (75th percentile for staple foods), and the maximum frequency of consumption (upper constraint of servings/week), both as the 90th percentile of reported intake and as adjusted to allow for an "added meal" per day in the Optifood models. The median and maximum number of servings per week by food group, and food sub-group, are presented in Table S4. A total of 66 individual food items were reported as consumed by pregnant and/or lactating women. Of these, 30 and 34 of these foods were consumed by ≥5% of lactating and pregnant women, respectively; and FBR generated by Optifood modeling were restricted to these commonly consumed foods. Grains and grain products, dark green leafy vegetables (DGLV), vegetable oils and legumes (pulses) were principle components of the diet. Food items recorded as being available in at least 11 of the 55 market surveys completed are presented in Table S5. In general, there were limited seasonal differences in availability and median prices. Of note, starchy roots, animal source foods, particularly meat, fish and eggs, and fruits were available in markets, but were rarely consumed by pregnant and lactating women (cumulatively <0.5% of eating occasions), and median serving sizes among consumers were small (e.g., meat, 34 g and egg, 64 g). Median prices per 100 g edible portions of animal source foods, excluding dairy, ranged from 0.22–0.47 €, compared to 0.03–0.10 € for grains and grain products.

3.2.2. Linear Programming

Reported Diet and Food-based Recommendations

Based on reported dietary intakes among pregnant and lactating women, the nutritionally "best" diets, with and without adherence to dietary food patterns (Module II), indicated that only zinc and iron reached >100% of the RDA (Tables S6 and S7). Linear programming analyses indicated that it was difficult to select a diet that achieved RDAs for all but three (vitamin B_6, iron and zinc) of the modeled micronutrients (Module III maximized diets where the best-case scenario is > 100% of the RDA; Tables 4 and 5). The remaining eight micronutrients that were modeled were identified as "problem" nutrients and likely to remain inadequate among this population, given the local food supply and food patterns. Thus, model constraints were changed prior to selecting (Module II) and testing (Module III) FBRs for these women (see below). Among pregnant women, including daily iron and folic acid supplements as the standard-of-care practice would ensure a low percentage of women would be at risk of inadequate intakes of folate, in addition to the already adequate intakes of iron, vitamin B_6 and zinc, but would do nothing to alleviate the remaining micronutrient inadequacies.

"Added Meal" and Food-Based Recommendations

Since observed mean energy intakes were substantially less than EER, scenarios were modeled which included the provision of an "added meal" per day (Tables 1 and S3). In Module II, the nutritionally "best" diet without considering current food patterns achieved 100% of the RDA for seven micronutrients among pregnant women and six micronutrients among lactating women, indicating at least one modelled diet can achieve RDAs for these nutrients (Tables S6 and S7). Final sets of FBR were selected (Table 6), with and without IFA supplements for pregnant women, which resulted in worst-case scenario values >65% of the RDA for thiamin, riboflavin, B_6, folate, iron, zinc and calcium for both pregnant and lactating women, plus vitamin A for pregnant women only (Tables 4 and 5). However, even if the set of FBR was successfully adopted, vitamins B_{12}, C and niacin values were < 65% of the RDA indicating the FBRs would not ensure a low percentage of pregnant and lactating women would be at risk of inadequate intakes for these nutrients. In addition, vitamin A values were < 65% of the RDA in lactating women, due to higher dietary recommendations. The minimum cost of a diet including an added meal per day, combined with FBR, was estimated to be 0.43 €/day for both pregnant and lactating women.

Table 4. The nutrient content of worst-case and best-case scenario diets without food-based recommendations (module III), and food-based recommendations with the greatest nutritional impact expressed as a percentage of Recommended Dietary Allowances (RDA) among pregnant women [1,2].

Analysis [3]	% of RDA											No. MN Adequate	Cost of Diet (€/day)
	Vitamin A	Vitamin C	Thiamin	Riboflavin	Niacin	Vitamin B6	Folate	Vitamin B12	Iron	Zinc	Calcium [4]		
Reported energy intake													
Best-case scenario	79.2	39.6	82.7	78.9	57.6	113.0	70.6	24.7	133.4	177.2	53.5	3	
Worst-case scenario	0	0.1	38.6	23.3	27.9	50.2	7.1	1.8	32.9	78.8	2.4	1	
Reported energy intake + IFA													
Best-case scenario	79.2	39.6	83.4	79.6	57.6	113.5	184.1	25.0	355.9	177.3	53.5	4	
Worst-case scenario	0	0.1	39.3	24.0	27.9	50.7	120.3	2.1	254.8	78.9	2.4	3	
Added meal													
Best-case scenario	111.8	65.6	122.6	121.9	87.0	154.9	116.6	47.1	188.2	267.7	87.4	7	
Worst-case scenario	0	0.1	50.5	25.7	38.1	62.8	9.9	2.4	32.8	100.1	1.4	1	
Best modeled FBR (worst-case scenario)	74.5	26.3	77.5	80.9	52.5	107.4	73.9	39.8	106.7	209.9	66.4	8	0.43
Added meal + IFA													
Best-case scenario	111.8	65.6	123.3	122.7	87.1	155.4	230.1	47.4	410.8	267.8	87.4	7	
Worst-case scenario	0	0.1	51.2	26.4	38.1	63.4	123.1	2.7	254.7	100.2	1.4	3	
Best modeled FBR (worst-case scenario)	74.4	26.1	70.6	79.9	52.2	106.3	167.3	40.0	323.7	205.2	65.1	8	0.42
Added meal + UNIMMAP													
Best-case scenario	215.8	148.0	222.7	222.1	187.2	255.1	230.1	147.2	299.5	404.2	87.4	10	
Worst-case scenario	103.8	82.3	150.3	125.6	137.9	162.7	123.1	102.2	143.8	236.3	1.4	10	
Best modeled FBR (worst-case scenario)	134.1	108.3	169.8	179.0	152.0	205.6	167.3	139.5	212.7	341.3	65.1	11	0.40
Added meal + Supercereal (CSB+)													
Best-case scenario	239.1	151.4	146.3	221.0	132.8	204.6	135.9	123.5	208.3	300.7	136.8	11	
Worst-case scenario	142.4	85.9	73.6	131.1	86.0	117.3	30.1	78.9	66.6	139.9	51.7	9	
Best modeled FBR (worst-case scenario)	152.6	100.5	86.7	140.5	89.9	128.3	71.1	79.2	78.7	145.9	68.9	11	0.19
Added meal + SQ-LNS P & L													
Best-case scenario	215.8	183.4	319.4	319.5	284.9	349.5	229.1	247.2	259.5	532.0	115.0	11	
Worst-case scenario	103.8	117.5	245.5	223.7	235.5	256.8	122.1	201.9	103.9	362.6	29.1	10	
Best modeled FBR (worst-case scenario)	128.0	141.8	248.0	248.5	244.7	278.6	126.9	220.5	112.5	396.6	71.1	11	0.28
Added meal + Plumpy'Mum													
Best-case scenario	226.3	149.2	218.4	221.0	193.1	236.4	243.1	145.7	293.2	384.2	96.7	10	
Worst-case scenario	114.3	83.5	142.3	129.7	144.3	144.5	136.4	100.7	149.5	217.3	11.3	10	
Best modeled FBR (worst-case scenario)	144.5	109.0	146.9	164.3	157.8	166.5	142.2	137.7	158.2	287.3	68.6	11	0.30

[1] CSB+, corn soy blend plus; IFA, iron and folic acid supplement; MN, micronutrients; SQ-LNS, small-quantity lipid-based nutrient supplement; P&L, pregnancy and lactation. [2] Best case scenario: diets sequentially modeled for each micronutrient, which would provide the highest possible amount (expressed as % of the RDA) of that micronutrient. "Problem" nutrients (non-shaded) were defined as nutrients where the nutrient did not achieve 100% of the RDA in the maximized best-case scenario; these are nutrients that will likely remain inadequate in the population given the local food supply and food patterns, even if women were to follow the FBR. Worst-case scenario: diets sequentially modeled for each micronutrient, which would provide the least possible amount (expressed as % of the RDA) of that micronutrient. Dietary adequacy for each nutrient was defined as the worst-case scenario for that nutrient being > 65% of the RDA (shaded); if the worst-case scenario is less than 65% (non-shaded) of the RDA, the nutrient is likely to be inadequate in the population, given local food supply and food patterns. [3] Energy constraints, food serving sizes and food consumption patterns are presented in Tables 1 and 4, and Supplemental Tables S1–S3. Best-modeled FBR are presented in Table 6 for each series. [4] Series modeled using calcium RDA of 1000 mg/day.

Table 5. The nutrient content of worst-case and best-case scenario diets without food-based recommendations (module III), and food-based recommendations with the greatest nutritional impact, expressed as a percentage of Recommended Dietary Allowances (RDA) among lactating women [1,2].

Analysis [3]	% of RDA												
	Vitamin A	Vitamin C	Thiamin	Riboflavin	Niacin	Vitamin B6	Folate	Vitamin B12	Iron	Zinc	Calcium [4]	No. MN Adequate	Cost of Diet (€/day)
Current energy intake													
Best-case scenario	52.3	40.9	95.4	83.3	72.3	128.0	81.7	21.9	245.1	199.8	54.8	3	
Worst-case scenario	0.0	0.0	51.9	29.8	38.0	64.2	11.0	2.1	82.0	96.5	4.0	2	0.43
Additional meal													
Best-case scenario	80.9	67.4	128.0	118.5	97.8	155.3	135.3	40.7	306.4	270.7	89.0	6	
Worst-case scenario	0.0	0.1	53.2	25.4	42.1	61.5	11.7	2.4	59.9	98.1	1.9	1	
Best modeled FBR (worst-case scenario)	13.7	15.1	78.4	69.3	56.7	111.6	69.9	37.0	181.9	207.2	65.4	7	0.43
Additional meal + UNIMMAP													
Best-case scenario	142.6	125.8	228.1	206.1	203.9	250.5	271.4	133.7	473.3	395.9	89.0	10	
Worst-case scenario	61.5	58.3	153.0	112.8	147.8	156.3	147.5	95.1	226.3	222.9	1.9	8	
Best modeled FBR (worst-case scenario)	75.2	73.3	178.2	156.7	162.4	206.5	205.7	129.7	348.3	332.0	65.4	11	0.43
Additional meal + Supercereal (CSB+)													
Best-case scenario	156.4	128.2	151.9	204.7	146.1	201.8	158.3	111.7	325.7	300.3	138.4	11	
Worst-case scenario	84.5	60.8	80.9	117.5	93.8	116.5	37.5	73.4	111.2	139.1	51.9	8	
Best modeled FBR (worst-case scenario)	88.9	69.7	91.3	123.6	97.1	129.1	74.6	73.6	125.2	143.3	69.7	11	0.21
Additional meal + SQ-LNS P & L													
Best-case scenario	142.6	150.9	324.8	291.1	307.4	340.1	270.3	226.6	406.9	513.0	116.6	11	
Worst-case scenario	61.5	83.3	249.5	198.4	251.2	246.3	146.8	187.7	166.5	340.6	29.4	9	
Best modeled FBR (worst-case scenario)	71.5	96.9	251.7	213.3	259.9	265.1	150.4	204.8	174.9	372.5	69.9	11	0.30
Additional meal + Plumpy'Mum													
Best-case scenario	148.8	126.7	224.5	204.9	210.3	232.5	287.0	132.3	454.0	377.5	98.2	10	
Worst-case scenario	67.7	59.1	149.8	116.2	155.3	143.2	165.1	93.7	235.0	209.3	11.5	9	
Best modeled FBR (worst-case scenario)	81.3	73.7	153.0	139.6	168.6	162.4	169.5	128.0	243.4	274.0	67.3	11	0.32

[1] CSB+, corn soy blend plus; IFA, iron and folic acid supplement; MN, micronutrients; SQ-LNS, small-quantity lipid-based nutrient supplement; P&L, pregnancy and lactation. [2] Best case scenario: diets sequentially modeled for each micronutrient, which would provide the highest possible amount (expressed as % of the RDA) of that micronutrient. "Problem" nutrients (non-shaded) were defined as nutrients where the nutrient did not achieve 100% of the RDA in the maximized best-case scenario; these are nutrients that will likely remain inadequate in the population given the local food supply and food patterns, even if women were to follow the FBR. Worst-case scenario: diets sequentially modeled for each micronutrient, which would provide the least possible amount (expressed as % of the RDA) of that micronutrient. Dietary adequacy for each nutrient was defined as the worst-case scenario for that nutrient being > 65% of the RDA (shaded); if the worst-case scenario is less than 65% (non-shaded) of the RDA, the nutrient is likely to be inadequate in the population, given local food supply and food patterns. [3] Energy constraints, food serving sizes and food consumption patterns are presented in Tables 1 and 4, and Supplemental Tables S1–S3. Best-modeled FBR are presented in Table 6 for each series. [4] Series modeled using calcium RDA of 1000 mg/day.

Table 6. Food-based recommendations for pregnant and lactating women, by model series and intervention product [1].

	Pregnant Women	No. MN Adequate [2]	Lactating Women	No. MN Adequate
Reported diet [3]	—		—	
Reported diet + IFA (standard of care)	—		—	
Added meal diet	• 21 servings of DGLV • 14 servings of milk • 21 servings of cooked beans/lentils/peas • 14 servings of millet • 21 servings of vitamin A fortified vegetable oil	8	• 21 servings of DGLV • 14 servings of milk • 21 servings of cooked beans/lentils/peas • 14 servings of millet	7
Added meal diet + IFA	• 21 servings of DGLV • 14 servings of milk • 21 servings of cooked beans/lentils/peas • 14 servings of millet • 21 servings of vitamin A fortified vegetable oil	8	—	
Added meal diet + UNIMMAP	• 21 servings of DGLV • 14 servings of milk • 21 servings of cooked beans/lentils/peas • 14 servings of millet	11	• 21 servings of DGLV • 14 servings of milk • 21 servings of cooked beans/lentils/peas • 14 servings of millet	11
Added meal diet + Supercereal (CSB+)	• 14 servings of DGLV • 14 servings of cooked beans/lentils/peas	11	• 14 servings of DGLV • 14 servings of cooked beans/lentils/peas	11
Added meal + SQ-LNS (P&L)	• 21 servings of DGLV • 7 servings of milk	11	• 21 servings of DGLV • 7 servings of milk	11
Added meal diet + Plumpy'Mum	• 21 servings of DGLV • 14 servings of milk	11	• 21 servings of DGLV • 14 servings of milk	11

[1] CSB+, corn soy blend plus; DGLV, dark green leafy vegetables; IFA, iron and folic acid supplement; MN, micronutrients; SQ-LNS, small-quantity lipid-based nutrient supplement; P&L, pregnancy and lactation; —, not available. [2] Maximum number of micronutrients with the potential to be adequate, $n = 11$. [3] Reported diet: model energy constraint equal to the reported mean energy intake for each target group; Added meal diet: model energy constraint increased above the reported diet to approximate the provision of an "added meal" (~600 kcal) per day among pregnant women or to match estimated energy requirements in lactating women, in addition to the best set of food-based recommendations.

When rarely consumed nutrient-dense animal source foods were included in the models along with the aforementioned FBR (e.g., one egg/day or 100 g meat/day), no model was able to ensure women were at low risk of inadequate intakes for all micronutrients; vitamins B$_{12}$, C, and niacin remained <65% of the RDA in one or more models (Table S8). In addition, the estimated cost of the diet increased by 35–59% in comparison to modeled diets providing one added meal per day and including the best set of FBR.

Intervention Products and Food-based Recommendations

FBRs with the provision of an added meal, with or without IFA for pregnant women or the inclusion of a rarely consumed nutrient-dense food did not ensure that a low percentage of pregnant or lactating women were at risk of inadequate intakes for all micronutrients, therefore additional supplementation strategies were modeled (Table 1). Consuming one added meal per day, plus a UNIMMAP supplement or a food-based product (SQ-LNS P&L, Plumpy'Mum and Supercereal, would ensure that a low percentage of pregnant and lactating women would be at low risk of inadequate intakes for almost all modeled micronutrients with the consistent exception of calcium (Tables 4 and 5). Specific sets of FBR to complement each intervention product focused on calcium-rich food sources, including DGLV, fermented milk, pulses and/or millet (Table 6). When lower calcium recommendations were used (775–800 mg/day vs. 1000 mg/day), the provision of Plumpy'Mum reduced the need for fermented milk to be included in FBR, and the provision of SQ-LNS eliminated it (Tables S9–S11). Including intervention products, with FBR in the modeled diets, decreased the estimated cost of the diets, as models did not account for costs associated with the products themselves or programmatic implementation (Tables 4 and 5).

4. Discussion

The present analyses indicated that energy intakes in pregnant and lactating women in rural Zinder, Niger were low compared to their estimated energy requirements, which is corroborated by the finding of a high prevalence of undernutrition in the population. Additionally, analysis of usual dietary intakes indicated that the prevalence of inadequate micronutrient intake was greater than 50% for eight and nine of the eleven micronutrients evaluated, among lactating and pregnant women respectively. Similarly, a 2010 systematic review reporting micronutrient intake among women in resource-poor settings concluded that inadequate intakes of multiple micronutrients were common, with reported mean or median intakes in over 50% of the studies below the EAR [3]. In addition, these present findings are supported by recently published data on biochemical micronutrient status among pregnant women in the same population, which indicated that approximately 25–50% of women had low plasma concentrations of zinc, folate and vitamin B$_{12}$, and iron deficiency, and >75% had marginal vitamin A status and anemia [6].

Only one in six women reported adequate dietary diversity, consuming at least five of ten defined food groups the previous day and night. Initial Optifood analyses, based on reported diets, revealed it would be difficult to meet nutrient recommendations given current dietary patterns, unless energy intakes were increased. A second series of analyses, based on the recommendation to include one added meal per day, indicated that an increased caloric intake plus FBR to increase the weekly consumption of nutrient-dense foods (e.g., DGLV, dairy and legumes), could improve the nutritional quality of the diet. However, even if women adhered to the best set of FBR modeled in these analyses, FBR alone, with or without IFA supplements included as standard antenatal care, could not ensure that a low percentage of pregnant or lactating women would be at low risk of inadequate intake for all 11 micronutrients modeled. Dietary adequacy could not be ensured for vitamins A, C, B$_{12}$ and niacin. In general, nutrient-dense foods were either not commonly consumed (i.e., meat, fish and eggs, vitamin C-rich fruits and vegetables) and thus did not appear as options for inclusion in the FBR, or were consumed in insufficient quantities to meet dietary recommendations (vitamin A-rich DGLV and fortified vegetable oils).

Numerous linear programming analyses in other low-income settings have indicated the potential of FBR and locally available foods to improve dietary micronutrient adequacy among the infants and young children although in most settings combinations of FBR with fortified foods or dietary supplements would be required [15,16,18,47,50]. Among women of reproductive age in low income countries, linear programming analyses have indicated that in some instances micronutrient adequacy may be achievable with FBRs, when nutrient-dense foods are included that are typically infrequently consumed, (e.g., animal source foods such as liver and small fish) [42,49,51]. Similar to our findings, other studies have concluded that a modest set of FBR, in combination with micronutrient or food-based supplements, would be necessary to meet nutrient adequacy among women of reproductive age, or might be more feasible and acceptable than FBR alone [42,47].

The present study is a modeling analysis based on reported dietary intakes, and does not present results from an efficacy or effectiveness trial. Thus, it is not possible to make strong conclusions about the feasibility of different proposed solutions in the present study. For example, when modeling IFA supplements as a dietary supplement, 100% coverage and full adherence was assumed. However, in reality the coverage and the adherence are much lower. Among pregnant women enrolled in the baseline survey of the NiMaNu Project (*n* = 923), only 44% had received IFA supplements during their current pregnancy, and 69% of these women reported adherence to IFA supplementation as recommended (i.e., consumed IFA daily in the previous week) [21]. Nevertheless, this research does highlight the critical necessity of additional interventions in this population, and provides general guidelines for proposed solutions. FBR without monetary support, rations or the inclusion of supplements, would require large changes to current dietary patterns (increased caloric consumption particularly among pregnant women, consumption of nutrient-dense foods including dairy and animal-protein foods, etc.) that may not be feasible, considering household resource constraints and food consumptions patterns during pregnancy and lactation. Thus, the recommendation to include one additional meal per day, as recommended in the Essential Nutrition Actions [46], in addition to a set of FBR, may be difficult in this context, particularly for pregnant women.

In the present study, >50% of women were moderately to severely food insecure, and 68% were below the national poverty line, based on daily food consumption expenditures alone (0.44 €) [52]. Therefore, increasing the median daily cost of the diet from 0.37 € (0.30, 0.49) to a projected *minimum* cost of 0.43 €/day, may be cost-prohibitive for the majority of women, where food expenditures are already accounting for >50% of total expenditures and the consumption aggregate poverty line (food and non-food expenditures) is 0.67 €/day [52]. The Prospective Urban Rural Epidemiology Study examined availability and affordability of fruits and vegetables in 18 countries, and reported that households in low-income countries (Bangladesh, India, Pakistan and Zimbabwe) would have to spend >50% of their household income to purchase two servings of fruits and three servings of vegetables per individual per day (compared to 2% of household income in high-income countries) [53]. Market surveys indicated that multiple nutrient-dense foods including meat, fish and eggs, fruits and vitamin A- and C-rich vegetables were available in local and regional markets, irrespective of season. However, these foods were not commonly consumed, as reported on 24 h dietary recalls. Thus, although availability and access, particularly at the village level, may be barriers to consumption, decisions regarding dietary intake may also be driven by cost or food preferences based on taste, convenience and storage capabilities [42]. In a recent longitudinal qualitative study to assess the determinants of dietary practices during pregnancy in a neighboring region of rural Niger, pregnant women noted physiological, household, community and structural level constraints to consuming their ideal pregnancy diets (e.g., maternal morbidity and food aversions, limited financial autonomy of women regarding household food purchasing, limited supply of preferred food items in local markets and systemic poverty) [54].

Combining the provision of balanced protein-energy supplementation with food-based recommendations may ensure that a low percentage of women would be at risk of inadequate nutrient intakes, with projected minimum per capita diet costs of 0.19–0.32 €/day. However, even adherence to

FBR combined with supplementation products may be difficult for women to achieve. For example, most FBR relied heavily on the consumption of fermented milk (7–14 servings/week; equivalent to ~100–200 mL per day) to meet calcium requirements. Adhering to these FBR may be challenging, as currently, only 25% of pregnant and lactating women reported consuming fermented milk in their 24 h dietary recalls, and 90% reported consuming <7 servings/week. Alternative interventions include the provision of comprehensive "food baskets", containing both commodities and nutrient-dense foods, cash transfers, for pregnant and lactating women to purchase nutrient-dense foods at local markets, or homestead food production. However, these scenarios do not include any production or distribution costs for the supplemental products, food baskets or cash transfers and assume that all costs would be borne by the governmental or non-governmental organizations rather than the target population. In all proposed solutions, well designed and implemented behavior change interventions would be necessary to evaluate adherence to food-based recommendations and supplementation among pregnant and lactating women and further research would be necessary to evaluate feasibility and acceptability.

Optifood models rely on assumptions regarding dietary requirements and the accuracy of nutrient composition data. Previous research has shown that varying assumptions regarding nutrient requirements, bioavailability and absorption, and the nutrient composition of foods affects estimated global prevalences of inadequate micronutrient intake [30]. Of note, iron and zinc were not identified as problem nutrients in the present study, despite prevalences of iron deficiency (low ferritin and high soluble transferrin receptor) and low plasma zinc concentrations ranging from 21–41% among pregnant women in the same study area [6]. Given the documented deficiencies in these micronutrients through biochemical assessments, it may be prudent to interpret the modeling results with caution. Recommended dietary allowances for iron and zinc in pregnant and lactating women were based on those established by the FNB/IOM; iron RDA assumed 25% and 10% absorption, respectively, and zinc RDA assumed 27% and 38% absorption, respectively [3,37]. Given the predominantly plant-based diets of the study participants, variable fermentation practices and limited data on the phytate content of common foods, it is possible that iron and zinc bioavailability, and thus absorption, were lower than estimated, thus increasing dietary intake requirements. Finally, these analyses do not account for the conversion of tryptophan to niacin, which should be taken into account in the context of purported inadequate niacin intakes. However, in spite of all these uncertainties in specific micronutrient recommendations, linear programming of various scenarios consistently indicated that overall, pregnant and lactating women in this population have difficulty meeting nutrient recommendations, given locally available foods and food patterns.

The present study had several strengths and weaknesses. Estimations of usual intakes and development of FBR through linear programming rely on the quality of the dietary data collected. This study used quantitative 24 h dietary recall data, which is subject to omissions, under- or- over-reporting of consumption and inaccuracies in portion size estimates. To minimize errors and bias, an interactive, systematic multi-pass method, developed specifically for use in rural populations in low-income countries with low rates of literacy, was used [26]. Certified midwives were hired as fieldworkers and were rigorously trained and supervised in data collection. Prior to the recall day, participants received training in portion size estimation, standard dishware and pictorial memory-aide charts. In addition, numerous methods were employed to estimate portion size, including pre-prepared staple foods, standard dishware and household utensils and purchase price of foods bought outside the home. In spite of these precautions, it is likely that recalls were subject to inaccuracies in reporting. In addition, estimates also depend on the accuracy and validity of food composition tables. Nutrient composition data are limited for locally available and wild food items, and it is difficult to account for the retention and bioavailability of nutrients in home-processed foods (e.g., milled, fermented, dried, cooked, etc.). Models assumed universal fortification of vegetable oils and wheat flour per national policy; however, the true extent of coverage is unknown. In addition, all bouillon cubes were assumed to be fortified with iron, but fortification is voluntary and not practiced by all producers. If vegetable oils, wheat flour or bouillon cubes consumed by this population are unfortified, or micronutrient retention in fortified products is low, vitamin A, iron and folate may be more likely to be problem nutrients than it appeared in these analyses. Finally, these analyses were limited to the micronutrients for which there are reference data available in the Optifood software; analysis of the micronutrient adequacy of additional micronutrients would be of interest.

5. Conclusions

In summary, linear programming of various scenarios consistently indicated that overall, pregnant and lactating women in this population have difficulty meeting nutrient recommendations given locally available foods and dietary patterns. Providing IFA supplements to pregnant women as the current standard of care in this population is inadequate to address multi-micronutrient inadequacies. In addition, modeling possible FBR suggests that these would not adequately address micronutrient deficiencies and may be cost-prohibitive for the local context. Thus, multiple micronutrient supplementation, and the provision of nutrient-dense food-based interventions should be considered. Effectiveness trials and program implementation research will be instrumental to determine the likelihood of various scenarios (sets of FBR and multiple micronutrient or balanced protein-energy supplements) to improve micronutrient intakes and biochemical and functional nutritional status.

Supplementary Materials: The following are available online at http://www.mdpi.com/2072-6643/11/1/72/s1, Table S1: Nutrient composition of intervention products modeled using the Optifood software tool, Table S2: Recommended Dietary Allowances (RDA) used for analyses, Table S3: Food serving size (g/day) and food consumption patterns (number of servings per week by percentiles) in pregnant and lactating study participants, Table S4: Consumption patterns of food group and food subgroup (number of servings per week by percentiles) in pregnant and lactating study participants, Table S5: Market availability and prices of foods from 55 markets surveys conducted at 10 markets in the study area over a period of 18 months, Table S6: The nutrient content of optimal diets with and without considering reported food patterns (module II), expressed as a percentage of Recommended Dietary Allowances (RDA) among pregnant women, Table S7: The nutrient content of optimal diets with and without food patterns (module II), expressed as a percentage of Recommended Dietary Allowances (RDA) among lactating women, Table S8: The nutrient content of worst-case and best-case scenario diets without food-based recommendations (module III), and food-based recommendations with the greatest nutritional impact expressed as a percentage of Recommended Dietary Allowances (RDA) among pregnant and lactating women, Table S9: The nutrient content of worst-case and best-case scenario diets without food-based recommendations (module III), and food-based recommendations with the greatest nutritional impact expressed as a percentage of Recommended Dietary Allowances (RDA) among pregnant women, using lower calcium recommendations (775 mg/day), Table S10: The nutrient content of worst-case and best-case scenario diets without food-based recommendations (module III), and food-based recommendations with the greatest nutritional impact expressed as a percentage of Recommended Dietary Allowances (RDA) among lactating women, using lower calcium recommendations (800 mg/day), Table S11: Food-based recommendations for pregnant and lactating women using lower calcium recommendations (775–800 mg/day), by model series and intervention product.

Author Contributions: Conceptualization, K.R.W., C.T.O. and S.Y.H.; Data curation, K.R.W. and R.R.Y.; Formal analysis, K.R.W. and R.R.Y.; Funding acquisition, K.R.W. and S.Y.H.; Investigation, C.T.O. and M.T.F.; Methodology, K.R.W., R.R.Y., E.L.F., C.T.O. and S.Y.H.; Project administration, K.R.W., C.T.O., M.T.F. and S.Y.H.; Supervision, K.R.W., C.T.O., M.T.F. and S.Y.H.; Writing – original draft, K.R.W.; Writing – review & editing, R.R.Y., E.L.F., C.T.O., M.T.F. and S.Y.H.

Funding: This research was funded by Nutriset, SAS (Malauney, France), grant number 201503315, and the main Niger Maternal Nutrition Project with the financial support of the Government of Canada through Global Affairs Canada and Nutrition International, formerly the Micronutrient Initiative, grant number 201300662. The project described was supported by the National Center for Advancing Translational Sciences (NCATS), National Institutes of Health (NIH), grant number UL1 TR000002.

Acknowledgments: We thank Reina Engle-Stone (University of California, Davis, USA) and Sara E. Wuehler (Nutrition International, Canada) for sharing data collection tools and expertise.

Conflicts of Interest: C.T.O.: Nutriset SAS provided financial support for C.T.O. PhD dissertation. K.R.W., R.R.Y., E.L.F., M.T.F., S.Y.H.: The authors declare no conflict of interest. The funders had no role in the design of the study; in the collection, analyses, or interpretation of data; in the writing of the manuscript, or in the decision to publish the results.

Abbreviations

AMDR	acceptable macronutrient distribution range
CSB+	corn soy blend plus
DGLV	dark green leafy vegetables
DRI	dietary reference intake
EAR	estimated average requirement
ECVMA	National Survey on Living Conditions, Household and Agriculture
EER	estimated energy requirement
FBR	food based recommendation
FNB	Food and Nutrition Board
HFIAS	household food insecurity access scale
IFA	iron and folic acid
IOM	Institute of Medicine
MDD-W	minimum dietary diversity for women
MN	micronutrients
MUAC	mid-upper arm circumference
NCI	National Cancer Institute
NiMaNu	Niger Maternal Nutrition Project
PAL	physical activity level
RDA	recommended dietary allowance
SQ-LNS P&L	small quantity lipid-based nutrient supplement for pregnant and lactating women
UEMOA	West African Economic and Monetary Union
UNIMMAP	UNICEF/WHO/UNU international multiple micronutrient preparation
USDA	United States Department of Agriculture
USDA SR28	USDA Nutrient Database for Standard Reference, Release 28
WHO	World Health Organization

References

1. Black, R.E.; Victora, C.G.; Walker, S.P.; Bhutta, Z.A.; Christian, P.; De Onis, M.; Ezzati, M.; Grantham-McGregor, S.; Katz, J.; Martorell, R.; et al. Maternal and child undernutrition and overweight in low-income and middle-income countries. *Lancet* **2013**, *382*, 427–451. [CrossRef]
2. Dror, D.K.; Allen, L.H. Overview of nutrients in human milk. *Adv. Nutr.* **2018**, *9*, 278S–294S. [CrossRef] [PubMed]
3. Torheim, L.E.; Ferguson, E.L.; Penrose, K.; Arimond, M. Women in resource-poor settings are at risk of inadequate intakes of multiple micronutrients. *J. Nutr.* **2010**, *140*, 2051S–2058S. [CrossRef] [PubMed]
4. UNICEF. At a Glance: Niger. 2014. Available online: http://unicef.org/infobycountry/niger_statistics.html (accessed on 14 October 2014).
5. Ouedraogo, C.; Young, R.; Wessells, K.; Hess, S. Prevalence and determinants of inadequate gestational weight gain among pregnant women in Zinder, Niger. *Curr. Dev. Nutr.* **2018**, in press.
6. Wessells, K.R.; Ouedraogo, C.T.; Young, R.R.; Faye, M.T.; Brito, A.; Hess, S.Y. Micronutrient status among pregnant women in Zinder, Niger and risk factors associated with deficiency. *Nutrients* **2017**, *9*. [CrossRef]
7. Institut National de la Statistique du Niger et Banque Mondiale. Profil et Determinants de la Pauvrete au Niger en 2011. Premiers Resultats de l'enquete Nationale sur les Conditions de vie: Des Menages et l'agriculture au Niger (ECVMA). 2013. Available online: http://www.stat-niger.org/statistique/file/Annuaires_Statistiques/Profil_Pauvrete_2011_ECVMA.pdf (accessed on 6 March 2015).
8. Imdad, A.; Bhutta, Z.A. Effect of balanced protein energy supplementation during pregnancy on birth outcomes. *BMC Public Health* **2011**, *11*, S17. [CrossRef]
9. Ramakrishnan, U.; Grant, F.K.; Imdad, A.; Bhutta, Z.A.; Martorell, R. Effect of multiple micronutrient versus iron-folate supplementation during pregnancy on intrauterine growth. *Nestle Nutr. Inst. Workshop Ser.* **2013**, *74*, 53–62. [CrossRef]
10. Ota, E.; Hori, H.; Mori, R.; Tobe-Gai, R.; Farrar, D. Antenatal dietary education and supplementation to increase energy and protein intake. *Cochrane Database Syst. Rev.* **2015**, *6*. [CrossRef]

11. Kaestel, P.; Michaelsen, K.F.; Aaby, P.; Friis, H. Effects of prenatal multimicronutrient supplements on birth weight and perinatal mortality: A randomised, controlled trial in Guinea-Bissau. *Eur. J. Clin. Nutr.* **2005**, *59*, 1081–1089. [CrossRef]

12. Adu-Afarwuah, S.; Lartey, A.; Dewey, K.G. Meeting nutritional needs in the first 1000 days: A place for small-quantity lipid-based nutrient supplements. *Ann. N. Y. Acad. Sci.* **2017**, *1392*, 18–29. [CrossRef]

13. The Sackler Institute for Nutrition Science. Nutrition Modeling Tools for Advocacy, Decision-Making and Costing: A Workshop to Support Adoption and Utilization. April 27–28, 2017. Available online: https://www.nyas.org/programs/the-sackler-institute-for-nutrition-science/evidence-based-tools-for-decision-making-in-nutrition-programs/ (accessed on 4 December 2018).

14. Ferguson, E.L.; Darmon, N.; Fahmida, U.; Fitriyanti, S.; Harper, T.B.; Premachandra, I.M. Design of optimal food-based complementary feeding recommendations and identification of key "problem nutrients" using goal programming. *J. Nutr.* **2006**, *136*, 2399–2404. [CrossRef] [PubMed]

15. Skau, J.K.; Bunthang, T.; Chamnan, C.; Wieringa, F.T.; Dijkhuizen, M.A.; Roos, N.; Ferguson, E.L. The use of linear programming to determine whether a formulated complementary food product can ensure adequate nutrients for 6- to 11-month-old Cambodian infants. *Am. J. Clin. Nutr.* **2014**, *99*, 130–138. [CrossRef] [PubMed]

16. Hlaing, L.M.; Fahmida, U.; Htet, M.K.; Utomo, B.; Firmansyah, A.; Ferguson, E.L. Local food-based complementary feeding recommendations developed by the linear programming approach to improve the intake of problem nutrients among 12-23-month-old Myanmar children. *Br. J. Nutr.* **2016**, *116*, S16–S26. [CrossRef] [PubMed]

17. Fahmida, U.; Santika, O.; Kolopaking, R.; Ferguson, E. Complementary feeding recommendations based on locally available foods in Indonesia. *Food Nutr. Bull.* **2014**, *35*, 174S–179S. [CrossRef] [PubMed]

18. Vossenaar, M.; Knight, F.A.; Tumilowicz, A.; Hotz, C.; Chege, P.; Ferguson, E.L. Context-specific complementary feeding recommendations developed using Optifood could improve the diets of breast-fed infants and young children from diverse livelihood groups in northern Kenya. *Public Health Nutr.* **2017**, *20*, 971–983. [CrossRef]

19. Tharrey, M.; Olaya, G.A.; Fewtrell, M.; Ferguson, E. Adaptation of new Colombian food-based complementary feeding recommendations using linear programming. *J. Pediatr. Gastroenterol. Nutr.* **2017**, *65*, 667–672. [CrossRef]

20. Hess, S.Y.; Ouedraogo, C.T. NiMaNu Project. Open Science Framework. 2016. Available online: Osf.io/4cenf (accessed on 30 June 2018).

21. Begum, K.; Ouedraogo, C.T.; Wessells, K.R.; Young, R.R.; Faye, M.T.; Wuehler, S.E.; Hess, S.Y. Prevalence of and factors associated with antenatal care seeking and adherence to recommended iron-folic acid supplementation among pregnant women in Zinder, Niger. *Mater. Child. Nutr.* **2018**, *14*. [CrossRef]

22. United Nations. Designing Household Survey Samples: Practical Guidelines. Available online: https://unstats.un.org/unsd/demographic/sources/surveys/Handbook23June05.pdf (accessed on 4 February 2014).

23. Coates, J.; Swindale, A.; Bilinksky, P. Household Food Insecurity Access Scale (HFIAS) for Measurement of Household Food Access: Indicator Guide (v. 3). Washington, D.C.: FHI 360/FANTA. Available online: https://www.fantaproject.org/monitoring-and-evaluation/household-food-insecurity-access-scale-hfias (accessed on 7 November 2013).

24. Ververs, M.T.; Antierens, A.; Sackl, A.; Staderini, N.; Captier, V. Which anthropometric indicators identify a pregnant woman as acutely malnourished and predict adverse birth outcomes in the humanitarian context? *PLoS Curr.* **2013**, *5*. [CrossRef]

25. Papageorghiou, A.T.; Ohuma, E.O.; Gravett, M.G.; Hirst, J.; Da Silveira, M.F.; Lambert, A.; Jaffer, Y.A.; Bertino, E.; Gravett, M.G.; Purwar, M.; et al. International standards for symphysis-fundal height based on serial measurements from the Fetal Growth Longitudinal Study of the INTERGROWTH-21st Project: Prospective cohort study in eight countries. *BMJ* **2016**, *355*, i5662. [CrossRef]

26. Gibson, R.; Ferguson, E. An Interactive 24-H Recall for Assessing the Adequacy of Iron and Zinc Intakes in Developing Countries. Harvest Plus Technical Monograph 8, 2002. Available online: http://www.harvestplus.org/node/544 (accessed on 17 October 2012).

27. FAO and FHI 360. *Minimum Dietary Diversity for Women: A Guide for Measurement*; FAO: Rome, Italy, 2016; Available online: http://www.fao.org/nutrition/assessment/tools/minimum-dietary-diversity-women/en/ (accessed on 25 May 2016).

28. Ministere de l'economie et des finances. Institut National de la Statistique. Troisieme Enquete Nationale sur le Budget et la Consommation des Menages au Niger. Manuel de l'enqueteur. 2007. Available online: http://catalog.ihsn.org/index.php/catalog/2300/download/36678 (accessed on 3 October 2013).

29. US Department of Agriculture, Agricultural Research Service, Nutrient Data Laboratory. USDA National Nutrient Database for Standard Reference, Release 28 (Slightly revised). Version Current: May 2016. Available online: http://www.ars.usda.gov/ba/bhnrc/ndl (accessed on 25 January 2017).

30. Wessells, K.R.; Singh, G.M.; Brown, K.H. Estimating the global prevalence of inadequate zinc intake from national food balance sheets: Effects of methodological assumptions. *PLoS ONE* **2012**, *7*, e50565. [CrossRef]

31. US Department of Agriculture. USDA table of nutrient retention factors, release 6. Available online: https://www.ars.usda.gov/ARSUserFiles/80400525/Data/retn/retn06.pdf (accessed on 1 May 2016).

32. *Portant application obligatoire des normes nigériennes relatives aux huiles comestibles raffinées de palme, palmiste et d'arachide enrichies en vitamine A*; Arrête conjoint N 65 MM/DI/MSP/MF du 25 Avril 2012; Ministère des Mines et du Développement Industriel, Ministère de la Santé Publique, Ministère des Finances: Niamey, République du Niger, 2012.

33. *Portant application obligatoire de la norme nigérienne relative à la farine de blé tendre enrichie en fer et acide folique*; Arrête conjoint N 89 MM/DI//MSP/MF du 31 Mai 2012; Ministère des Mines et du Développement Industriel, Ministère de la Santé Publique, Ministère des Finances: Niamey, République du Niger, 2012.

34. Food Fortification Initiative. Country Profile - Niger. Available online: http://ffinetwork.org/country_profiles/country.php?record=158 (accessed on 4 September 2018).

35. Luo, H.; Stewart, C.; Vosti, S.; Brown, K.; Engle-Stone, R. Predicted effects of current and potential micronutrient intervention programs on adequacy of iron intake in a national sample of women and young children in Cameroon. In Proceedings of the Micronutrient Forum, Cancun, Mexico, October 2016.

36. Institute of Medicine. *Food and Nutrition Board. Dietary Reference Intakes for Vitamin C, Vitamin E, Selenium and Carotenoids*; National Academy Press: Washington, DC, USA, 2000.

37. Institute of Medicine. *Food and Nutrition Board. Dietary Reference Intakes for Vitamin A, Vitamin K, Arsenic, Boron, Chromium, Iodine, Iron, Manganese, Molybdenum, Nickel, Silicon, Vanadium, and Zinc*; National Academy Press: Washington, DC, USA, 2001.

38. Institute of Medicine. Food and Nutrition Board. Dietary Reference Intakes for Calcium and Vitamin D. Available online: https://ods.od.nih.gov/Health_Information/Dietary_Reference_Intakes.aspx (accessed on 4 July 2018).

39. Institute of Medicine. Food and Nutrition Board. Dietary Reference Intakes for Energy, Carbohydrate, Fiber, Fat, Fatty Acids, Cholesterol, Protein, and Amino Acids. Available online: https://ods.od.nih.gov/Health_Information/Dietary_Reference_Intakes.aspx (accessed on 3 February 2010).

40. Institute of Medicine. *Food and Nutrition Board. Dietary Reference Intakes: Thiamin, Riboflavin, Niacin, Vitamin B6, Vitamin B12, Pantothenic Acid, Biotin, and Choline*; National Academy Press: Washington, DC, USA, 1998.

41. World Health Organization, Food and Agriculture Organization. *Vitamin and Mineral Requirements in Human Nutrition. Report of a Joint FAO/WHO Expert Consultation*; World Health Organization: Geneva, Switzerland, 2004.

42. Arimond, M.; Vitta, B.S.; Martin-Prevel, Y.; Moursi, M.; Dewey, K.G. Local foods can meet micronutrient needs for women in urban Burkina Faso, but only if rarely consumed micronutrient-dense foods are included in daily diets: A linear programming exercise. *Mater. Child. Nutr.* **2018**, *14*. [CrossRef]

43. Tooze, J.A.; Kipnis, V.; Buckman, D.W.; Carroll, R.J.; Freedman, L.S.; Guenther, P.M.; Krebs-Smith, S.M.; Subar, A.F.; Dodd, K.W. A mixed-effects model approach for estimating the distribution of usual intake of nutrients: The NCI method. *Stat. Med.* **2010**, *29*, 2857–2868. [CrossRef] [PubMed]

44. Tooze, J.A.; Midthune, D.; Dodd, K.W.; Freedman, L.S.; Krebs-Smith, S.M.; Subar, A.F.; Guenther, P.M.; Carroll, R.J.; Kipnis, V. A new statistical method for estimating the usual intake of episodically consumed foods with application to their distribution. *J. Am. Diet. Assoc.* **2006**, *106*, 1575–1587. [CrossRef] [PubMed]

45. Daelmans, B.; Ferguson, E.; Lutter, C.K.; Singh, N.; Pachon, H.; Creed-Kanashiro, H.; Woldt, M.; Mangasaryan, N.; Cheung, E.; Mir, R.; et al. Designing appropriate complementary feeding recommendations: Tools for programmatic action. *Mater. Child. Nutr.* **2013**, *9*, 116–130. [CrossRef] [PubMed]

46. Guyon, A.B.; Quinn, V.J. Booklet on Key Essential Nutrition Actions Messages. Available online: http://www.thp.org/files/Booklet_of_Key_ENA_Messages_complete_for_web.pdf (accessed on 14 January 2015).

47. FANTA. Development of Evidence-Based Dietary Recommendations for Children, Pregnant Women, and Lactating Women Living in the Western Highlands in Guatemala. 2014. Available online: https://www.fantaproject.org/countries/guatemala/optifood-report-2014 (accessed on 24 February 2015).

48. Santika, O.; Fahmida, U.; Ferguson, E.L. Development of food-based complementary feeding recommendations for 9- to 11-month-old peri-urban Indonesian infants using linear programming. *J. Nutr.* **2009**, *139*, 135–141. [CrossRef] [PubMed]

49. Levesque, S.; Delisle, H.; Agueh, V. Contribution to the development of a food guide in Benin: Linear programming for the optimization of local diets. *Public Health Nutr.* **2015**, *18*, 622–631. [CrossRef] [PubMed]

50. Termote, C.; Raneri, J.; Deptford, A.; Cogill, B. Assessing the potential of wild foods to reduce the cost of a nutritionally adequate diet: An example from eastern Baringo District, Kenya. *Food Nutr. Bull.* **2014**, *35*, 458–479. [CrossRef]

51. Biehl, E.; Klemm, R.D.; Manohar, S.; Webb, P.; Gauchan, D.; West, K.P., Jr. What does it cost to improve household diets in Nepal? Using the cost of the diet method to model lowest cost dietary changes. *Food Nutr. Bull.* **2016**, *37*, 247–260. [CrossRef]

52. World Bank. Republic of Niger: Measuring Poverty Trends. Available online: https://openknowledge.worldbank.org/handle/10986/22808 (accessed on 3 March 2018).

53. Miller, V.; Yusuf, S.; Chow, C.K.; Dehghan, M.; Corsi, D.J.; Lock, K.; Popkin, B.; Rangarajan, S.; Khatib, R.; Lear, S.A.; et al. Availability, affordability, and consumption of fruits and vegetables in 18 countries across income levels: Findings from the Prospective Urban Rural Epidemiology (PURE) study. *Lancet Glob. Health.* **2016**, *4*, e695–e703. [CrossRef]

54. Rosen, J.G.; Clermont, A.; Kodish, S.R.; Matar Seck, A.; Salifou, A.; Grais, R.F.; Isanaka, S. Determinants of dietary practices during pregnancy: A longitudinal qualitative study in Niger. *Mater. Child. Nutr.* **2018**, *14*, e12629. [CrossRef]

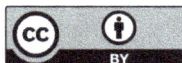

nutrients

MDPI

Review

Elemental Metabolomics and Pregnancy Outcomes

Daniel R. McKeating, Joshua J. Fisher and Anthony V. Perkins *

School of Medical Science, Menzies Health Institute Queensland, Griffith University, Southport 9726, Queensland, Australia; d.mckeating@griffith.edu.au (D.R.M.); josh.fisher@griffith.edu.au (J.J.F.)
* Correspondence: A.Perkins@griffith.edu.au; Tel.: +61-(0)-7-5552-9774; Fax: +61-(0)-7-5552-8908

Received: 19 November 2018; Accepted: 1 January 2019; Published: 2 January 2019

check for
updates

Abstract: Trace elements are important for human health and development. The body requires specific micronutrients to function, with aberrant changes associated with a variety of negative health outcomes. Despite this evidence, the status and function of micronutrients during pregnancy are relatively unknown and more information is required to ensure that women receive optimal intakes for foetal development. Changes in trace element status have been associated with pregnancy complications such as gestational diabetes mellitus (GDM), pre-eclampsia (PE), intrauterine growth restriction (IUGR), and preterm birth. Measuring micronutrients with methodologies such as elemental metabolomics, which involves the simultaneous quantification and characterisation of multiple elements, could provide insight into gestational disorders. Identifying unique and subtle micronutrient changes may highlight associated proteins that are affected underpinning the pathophysiology of these complications, leading to new means of disease diagnosis. This review will provide a comprehensive summary of micronutrient status during pregnancy, and their associations with gestational disorders. Furthermore, it will also comment on the potential use of elemental metabolomics as a technique for disease characterisation and prediction.

Keywords: elemental metabolomics; trace elements; pregnancy; micronutrition

1. Introduction

Biological trace elements are important for human health with imbalances in elemental homeostasis and metabolism playing a critical role in a variety of poor health outcomes. Micronutrition consists of elements required in small amounts in the daily diet that are essential for proper growth, development and physiology of organisms. For humans, this includes 13 elements that are not able to be synthesised, such as iron, selenium and calcium [1]. Recent studies suggest that, in some developed and relatively affluent societies, only 5% of the population meet the guidelines for adequate fruit and vegetable daily intake of 2 serves of fruit and 5 of vegetables, indicating that our diets may be lacking in essential nutrients that are principally acquired from these sources [2]. Maternal nutrition has long been considered to be important for a healthy pregnancy [3,4]. Adequate intake of macro nutrients has been correlated to positive pregnancy outcomes whereas hyperglycaemia, hyperlipidaemia and excessive calorific intakes have been associated with pregnancy complications. Similarly, the micronutrient status of women in many countries is below recommended daily intake (RDI) levels for both vitamins and minerals [5]. Due to the increasing demand for many micronutrients during pregnancy, the World Health Organization (WHO) recommends an increased intake of many nutrients during gestation and lactation [6]. Despite this, the global burden of maternal undernutrition including micronutrient deficiencies is persistent, particularly in South Asia where 10–40% are undernourished [7] Additionally, nutrients such as vitamin D, calcium, magnesium, and iron are consumed in quantities 74% lower than recommended levels in Australia; whilst vitamins A, C, and zinc consumption has been found to be 250% greater than recommendations, depending on the region [8].

Micronutrients play key roles in pregnancy outcomes, with aberrant micronutrition, such as deficiency in magnesium, potassium, calcium, selenium, and zinc being associated with poor perinatal outcomes such as gestational diabetes mellitus (GDM) and preeclampsia (PE), both are associated with an increase in other pregnancy complications including of fetal growth restriction (FGR), preterm birth and still birth [9,10]. Gestational disorders can lead to severe long term health outcomes for both mother and child after pregnancy, with this information in mind, it is of critical importance to identify women at risk of these complications as early in gestation as possible [11]. To limit the severity of negative outcomes or prevent disorders altogether, early detection and intervention is required.

The use of elemental metabolomics; the study of elements present within an organism, has only recently been developed to a point which might be applicable to understanding human health. Recent studies have successfully utilised trace element metabolomics to predict the onset and progression of Alzheimer's disease [12], Parkinson's disease [13], diabetes [14], and cancer [15]. Multi-elemental analysis and predictive capabilities of this methodology could contribute to further understand gestational disorders and possible use as a means of predicting pregnancy outcomes. Complexities surrounding nutrition and pregnancy are extensive with various elements correlated to diverse outcomes. Currently, only a handful of essential elements are known to affect pregnancy outcomes, even though there may be additional micronutrients that are essential for pregnancy health and human development [16].

2. Maternal Nutrition

The inadequate levels of micronutrients are well understood in low income countries [17]; however, there is surprisingly little known about the micronutrient status of pregnant women in many developed countries. Women often supplement their diet with multiple micronutrients during pregnancy, and many more may consume the high-fat, low-nutrient diets typical of high-income nations. Various micronutrients are important for successful pregnancy, although the specific pregnancy related functions of many are poorly understood. Sedentary lifestyle, tobacco smoking, alcohol consumption, and hypertension are maternal risk factors that have been extensively shown to cause an increased incidence of negative outcomes during gestation. Micronutrients have roles in modulation of the maternal and fetal metabolism, oxidative stress, placentation, and structural development of key fetal organs and tissues [3,4].

The placenta plays a crucial role in mediating the transfer of nutrients via both active and passive transport mechanisms [18]. Previous research indicates that the placenta will preferentially uptake nutrients from the maternal system to prevent fetal deficiency [19,20]. Maternal conditions such as diabetes or obesity can alter the nutrient transporters in the placenta, leading to increased or decreased nutritional flow, with potential outcomes including overgrowth (macrosomia) or intrauterine growth restriction (IUGR) of the foetus. As the placenta coordinates many aspects of gestational development and maternal blood nourishes the foetus, biological samples from the maternal or fetal circulation provide highly meaningful information relating to micronutrient status, maternal health and fetal development.

A concept popularised by David Barker known as "fetal programming" or the "Developmental Origins of Health and Disease" hypothesis, showed that there are a spectrum of processes that operate in all pregnancies and infancy that shape future health and risk of disease [21]. Fetal programming describes the maladaptive consequences to a maternal, fetal, or placental stressor during pregnancy that can result in abnormal development leading to disease [22].

Maternal nutrition has been specifically noted to have significant impacts on offspring outcome, as seen in the Dutch Famine (1944-45). After examining a cohort of 2414 people, it was noted that famine at any time during gestation was associated with glucose intolerance in offspring. If exposed early in gestation, there was an associated increase in obesity, coronary heart disease, atherogenic lipid profiles, disturbed blood coagulation, and increased stress responsiveness in offspring, while women who were conceived during this time had 5 times higher rates of breast cancer [23]. Although this study highlighted the complexities of human development, it also highlighted the importance of maternal nutrition and dietary profile of micro and macronutrition to the fetal environment. Though epidemiological studies have found correlations between over and under nutrition and programming of disease, few have managed to elucidate the mechanisms involved and the interrelationships of micronutrition in maternal and fetal health [24]. Currently, we only know how a selection of micronutrients affect pregnancy outcomes even though many additional micronutrients are likely to be essential to human development [16,25].

3. Micronutrition during Gestation and Lactation

3.1. Potassium

The RDI of potassium during pregnancy is 2800 mg/day to avoid deficiency (hypokalaemia) (Table 1). Potassium can be acquired from sources such as leafy green, root vegetables, beans, peas and fruits. Meat products, nuts and dairy products also have moderate amounts of potassium [16]. Normal blood concentration of potassium ranges from 14.1 to 20.3 mg/dL, with levels lower than 9.7 mg/dL indicative of hypokalaemia [26]. During pregnancy, birth outcomes based around hypokalaemia are unknown, however there is the possibility of negative maternal outcomes such as extreme muscle fatigue [27] or muscular paralysis [28]. Hypokalaemia is also concomitant with cardiac arrhythmias and muscle weakness [29,30]. Hyperkalaemia (high potassium) is often used as a marker of acute metabolic or renal dysfunction and has also been associated with severe atherosclerotic morbidity leading to cardiovascular disease. Similar to hypokalaemia, there is limited literature associating hyperkalaemia and poor pregnancy health, although both GDM and PE patients have a higher possibility to develop renal dysfunction [31].

Table 1. Recommended daily intake (RDI) and reference ranges for elements. Information gathered from Nutrient Reference Values for Australia and New Zealand. New Zealand Ministry of Health, 2006. [8], Gluckman, P., et al., Nutrition and lifestyle for pregnancy and breastfeeding. 2014: Oxford University Press, UK. [16], Farinde, A. Lab Values, Normal Adult: Laboratory Reference Ranges in Healthy Adults. Available online: https://emedicine.medscape.com/article/2172316-overview. [32], FSANZ. The 23rd Australian total diet study: Food Standards Australia New Zealand: 2011. [33]. Additional information from [34,35]. Elements that are not present did not have documented reference ranges. This is due to their normal concentration being unknown, or they are not in measurable quantities in human blood, serum, plasma, urine, or cord blood.

	RDI	Blood Reference Range	Serum/Plasma Reference Range	Urine Reference Range	Cord Reference Range
Na (Sodium)	460–920 mg [6]	310–335 mg/dL [36]	-	45 mg/dL [36]	290–380 mg/dL [36]
Mg (Magnesium)	350 mg [6]	3.6–6.1 mg/dL [36]	1.7–2.2 mg/dL [16]	145–245 mg/day [36]	-
P (Phosphorus)	1000 mg [6]	6–9.2 mg/dL [36]	2.7–4.4 mg/dL [36]	0.4–1.3 g/day [36]	-
S (Sulfur)	900 mg [6]	-	-	-	-
K (Potassium)	2800 mg [6]	14.1–20.3 mg/dL [36]	13.3–17.2 mg/dL [36]	97.7–490 mg/dL [36]	21.9–46.92 mg/dL [36]
Ca (Calcium)	1000 mg [6]	8.6–10.2 mg/dL [36]	8.6–10 mg/dL [36]	100–300mg/day [36]	-
V (Vanadium)	<1.8 mg [32]	-	<1 µg/L [36]	-	-
Cr (Chromium)	30 µg [6]	0.5–2.5 µg/L [33]	0.8–5.1 µg/mL [33]	-	-
Mn (Manganese)	5 mg [6]	4–15 µg/L [36]	0.4–0.85 µg/L [36]	1–8 µg/L [36]	-
Fe (Iron)	27 mg [6]	-	50–170 µg/dL [36]	-	-
Co (Cobalt)	-	0.7–3.4 µg/L [33]	0.3–7.5 µg/L [33]	-	-
Ni (Nickel)	-	-	<2 µg/L [36]	-	-
Cu (Copper)	1.3 mg [6]	70–140 µg/dL [36]	80–155 µg/dL [36]	3–35 µg/day [36]	4.6–8.8 µmol/L [34]
Zn (Zinc)	11 mg [6]	4.5–6.5 mg/L [36]	0.66–1.10 µg/mL [36]	5–50 µg/day [36]	15.8–22 µmol/L [34]
As (arsenic)	-	0.2–2.3 µg/dL [36]	-	-	-
Se (Selenium)	65 µg [6]	-	70–150 µg/L [36]	15–50 µg/L [36]	0.5–0.7 µmol/L [34]
Mo (Molybdenum)	50 µg [6]	0.6–4 µg/L [36]	0.3–2.0 µg/L [36]	-	-
I (Iodine)	220 µg [6]	-	40–92 µg/L [36]	150–249 µg/L [36]	-

3.2. Calcium

Daily calcium intake during pregnancy is recommended at 1000 mg/day, increasing to 1200 mg/day in the last trimester (Table 1), with Vitamin D also consumed along with calcium to allow for the adaptive homeostatic mechanisms for gestation and lactation to occur [6,37]. In western diets, milk and milk products are the primary sources of calcium; with cereals, fruits, and vegetables making a lesser contribution. Calcium's requirement by bone makes it critical during stages of rapid bone development, such as during gestation, infancy, childhood and adolescents [38]. Calcium is also important in the extracellular fluid for physiological function through mediation of cell signalling for both vasoconstriction, vasodilation, nerve transmission, contraction of muscles, and glandular secretion of hormones [38].

To maintain physiological functions within the body, calcium levels in the blood are maintained at around 8.6–10.2 mg/dL in adults, tightly controlled by the calcium sensing receptor, parathyroid hormone (PTH), and active vitamin D—1,25-Dihydroxyvitamin D [39]. Measurement of blood calcium is not an indication of total bone calcium, instead a representation of free calcium, a preferred indicator for those with protein abnormalities such as low albumin, which effects the ratio of free calcium vs. bound calcium. Measurements of calcium in urine are used to determine if renal excretion of calcium is normal. Serum concentration levels of calcium generally vary above or below the normal range under severe circumstances such as malnutrition or hyperparathyroidism [16]. When calcium levels decrease, the calcium sensing receptor triggers PTH release form the parathyroid gland which triggers the conversion of 25-hydroxyvitamin D to 1,25-Dihydroxyvitamin D, which increases circulating serum calcium levels from bone stores and increases smooth muscle contraction [39].

Low calcium levels are also concomitant with an increased release of renin from the kidneys, influencing maternal circulating renin-angiotensin-aldosterone systems (RAAS) leading to hypertension through vasoconstriction and fluid/sodium retention. The nonrenal renin-angiotensin systems (RAS) are important for ovulation, implantation, placentation, development of the uteroplacental, and umbilicoplacental circulation [40]. The function of the RAS in the maternal system is largely driven by maternal demand, and so the activity doesn't reflect the role of RAS in the placenta which may have other documented roles in pathological pregnancies such as IUGR, and PE [40]. Calcium supplementation has been shown to be associated with a reduction in the risk of gestational hypertensive disorders and an increase in birthweight [41].

3.3. Magnesium

The recommended intake of magnesium during pregnancy is 350 mg/day to maintain function of over 300 enzymes that utilise ATP (Table 1) [6,16]. Leafy green vegetables provide a good source of magnesium, due to its presence in the core of the chlorophyll molecule. Other important sources include whole grains, nuts, legumes, cereals, and seafood. Water can also be an important source of magnesium, dependant on how "Hard" or "Soft" the water, in hard water communities it can comprise up to 38% of the daily magnesium consumption [42]. Enzymes in energy metabolism and neuromuscular signalling require magnesium for substrate formation. Whilst acting as an allosteric activator for phospholipase C, adenylate cyclase, and Na/K-ATPase; magnesium also regulates calcium ion transport channels, calcium homeostasis, and is required for calcium-triggered release of PTH and PTH action [43].

There is no generally accepted measurement for adequate magnesium status, as 50 to 60% resides within bone [16]. Serum magnesium is the best measurement available, but only measures <1% of total body magnesium. The normal reference range for serum is between 1.7 to 2.2 mg/dL, with levels below 1.7 mg/dL often referred to as hypomagnesaemia [16,44]. There is currently no literature surrounding how reference ranges for circulating magnesium should be altered during gestation. Magnesium deficiency is often accompanied by calcium and potassium deficiencies. Calcium becomes deficient due to the impaired PTH secretion caused by low magnesium, causing a perpetuation of low serum calcium. The rise is active vitamin D to recruit calcium from the gut that is expected to follow is attenuated under calcium deficient conditions, propagating calcium deficiency. With potassium, magnesium is required for it to be adequately conserved by the kidneys. When magnesium is low, potassium levels cannot be maintained and can proceed to hypokalaemia [43,44]. There may be a neuro protective effect of high maternal magnesium intake on offspring, whilst also having positive effects on bone mineral density [30,45].

3.4. Manganese

Involved in cellular metabolic processes, manganese is a component of antioxidant enzymes such as superoxide dismutase, and essential for development and human health. The bioavailability of manganese is low, primarily consumed through whole grains, nuts, seeds, and tea [16,45–47]. Uptake and retention is dictated by dietary calcium, iron, and phosphorus [48,49]. To reach an adequate intake of manganese during pregnancy, it is recommended that 5 mg/day be consumed (Table 1) [6]. Manganese is a cofactor for an extensive number of enzymes, including oxidoreductases, transferases, hydrolases, lyases, isomerases, ligases, lectins, and integrins [50]. Two of its more important roles however are arginase, the last enzyme for the urea cycle, and the mitochondrial antioxidant manganese super oxide dismutase [50].

Normal levels of manganese in the body range from 4–15 μg/L in blood, 0.4–0.85 μg/L in serum, and 1–8 μg/L in urine [46]. Serum, plasma and urine concentrations have all been noted to respond to dietary manganese intake, leading to disagreement on the best indicator of status [51,52]. During pregnancy, manganese concentrations have been shown to increase over the course of gestation from 10–34 weeks, however values fit within the currently established reference ranges [53,54]. Recent studies examining excessive manganese exposure due to environmental pollution have suggested that excessive manganese levels in pregnancy can negatively impact on the cognitive develop of the unborn child [55]. Despite this, there is still a considerable need to investigate the effects of manganese on foetal development during gestation [16].

3.5. Iron

The RDI for iron is 27 mg/day, however analysis of women living in America has found that 90% will not meet 22 mg/day (Table 1). Iron enters the diet through two different forms, haem and non-haem. Haem is found within meats, poultry and fish due to the iron component in the oxygen-transport metalloprotein haemoglobin [56]. Alternatively, non-haem iron is found in cereals, legumes, fruits, and vegetables. Non-haem forms make up a larger portion of the diet, however are not as bioavailable as haem forms [57]. Serum iron levels range from 50–170 μg/dL for women, pregnancy iron levels increase to keep up with the haemoglobin levels of both mother and child, however they appear to drop in concentration because of increased blood volume. There are no serum iron reference ranges for pregnant women, though blood haemoglobin levels have been shown to decrease from 12–16 g/dL in non-pregnant to 10–14 g/dL in pregnancy [16].

Iron is required in a wide range of enzymes and pathways for its redox properties and coordination chemistry [58]. In mammals, iron is integral to cellular respiration, oxygen transport, energy production, and DNA synthesis [59]. Knowledge surrounding disease associated with iron revolves around the understanding of iron homeostasis. Levels of iron may be affected by various factors such as genetic variations, dietary influence, absorption, and haemolysis. Iron deficiency is the main cause of anaemia, resulting from iron's use in haemoglobin synthesis affecting healthy red blood cells [60]. High concentrations of iron within the blood can cause metabolic alterations resulting in increased incidence of insulin resistance and type 2 diabetes in pregnant women [30,61].

3.6. Copper

The adequate intake of copper for pregnancy is 1.3 mg/day, with the upper safe intake being 8–10 mg/day (Table 1) [6]. Serum or plasma total copper levels are around 60–140 μg/dL for a healthy adult, with no adequate reference range for pregnant women [16]. Copper is an essential element for fundamental biological functions such as accepting and donating electrons in oxidation-reduction reactions, oxidative phosphorylation, free-radical detoxification, neurotransmitter synthesis, and iron metabolism [62]. Sources of foodstuffs with high levels of copper include meats, shellfish, nuts, and cocoa products. Foodstuffs low in copper can also provide a significant amount to a person's intake, these include tea, potatoes, milk, and chicken [56].

Overnutrition of copper is mostly prevented during pregnancy by an emetic response, however can potentially result in toxic effects when over 15 mg are consumed [30]. Although there are no known associations with pregnancy overnutrition of copper, it has been considered a potential risk factor in cardiovascular disease [63,64]. High copper intake has also been negatively associated with cognitive function [65]. Undernutrition of copper is uncommon but can result from genetic uptake disorders or deficiency of trace elements from foodstuffs, more common in people consuming a Western diet [66]. Suboptimal intake in pregnancy may have negative effects on the developing lungs, skin, bones, organ systems and the immune system of the foetus. In newborns, copper deficiency manifests as oedema, anaemia, bone disease and recurrent apnoea [30,67]. Although copper is critical for pregnancy, supplementation is not recommended [16].

3.7. Zinc

Western diets meet the adequate daily intake of zinc for pregnant and lactating women of roughly 11 mg per day (Table 1) [16]. However, in analysis of upper and middle class households, it was found that greater than 30% of women did not reach this adequate intake level [68]. Zinc has both functional and structural roles in a number of enzyme systems that are important for gene expression, cell growth and division, neurotransmission, and reproductive and immune functions. A global search within the human genome has found that about 2800 proteins consist of a potential zinc binding site, making up around 10% of the proteome [69]. Shellfish, red meat, nuts, legumes, eggs, poultry, whole grains, some fruits and dairy products are all foodstuffs with a high bioavailability of zinc [16]. A meta-analysis by Foster, M. et al., (2015) on zinc status of vegetarians during pregnancy concluded that while vegetarian women have lower zinc intakes than non-vegetarian women, both groups consume lower than recommended amounts [70]. As a method of zinc status diagnosis, serum and plasma are used as a marker of deficiency with normal serum zinc levels ranging for 0.66–1.10 µg/mL [16].

Imbalances in zinc homeostasis are associated with a variety of human diseases. Often accompanied by malnourishment, zinc deficiency is estimated at 20–30% of the global population. Zinc is essential to physical and neurological development of infants and children, whilst also vital to protect plasma membranes from oxidative damage [71]. Immune system function is affected by zinc deficiency, increasing the risk and severity of infection [72]. Zinc also plays a significant role in neurological development of infants and children, with deficiency associated with neuronal atrophy, behavioural problems, and impaired cognitive development [16]. A number of poor gestational outcomes are associated with inadequate zinc intake. Zinc overnutrition is primarily associated with maternal gastrointestinal stress which has not been associated with poor maternal outcomes or fetal programming [16,30].

3.8. Iodine

The RDI for iodine is 220 µg/day during pregnancy (Table 1), however according to the WHO there is concern for iodine availability in areas around Europe, the Eastern Mediterranean, Africa, Himalayas, Andes, and Western Pacific [6,73]. Iodine is a key component of thyroid hormones, thyroxine (T4) and triiodothyronine (T3) which regulate growth, development, reproductive function, metabolic rate, cellular metabolism, and connective tissue integrity [74]. All biological actions of iodine are attributed to thyroid hormones. Seafoods and some dairy foodstuffs contain a large concentration of iodine. Whilst most iodine is derived from these sources, it is also possible to consume an adequate amount of iodine through eggs, meats, and bread [56]. Iodine is primarily excreted through urine and as a result is a good indicator of dietary iodine intake, with sufficiency defined as 150–249 µg/L [75].

Low iodine is correlated to impaired neurological development, in particular neuropsychological leading to cretinism, mental retardation and brain damage [30,76]. Attention Deficit Hyperactivity Disorder is also more common in offspring, this is believed to be due to the disruption of brain development and myelination of the central nervous system in utero [77]. Excess iodine intake has its own accompanying risks. Symptoms of acute toxicity involve diarrhoea, hyperactivity, weakness, convulsions, and possibly death [78]. Women with excessive iodine intakes are found to be more likely to be suffering from thyroid related diseases such as hypothyroidism resulting in maternal weight gain and haemolysis possibly resulting in negative fetal outcomes and death [79].

3.9. Selenium

Selenium is an essential trace element required in small amounts in the diet to comprise the primary component of selenoproteins that have various roles including antioxidant function [80]. It is recommended during pregnancy that women have an intake of 60 μg/day of selenium [81]. Food sources of selenium are affected by the soil content in which they are grown so in areas with proficient selenium in the soil there is a greater intake. Also, areas with high levels of sulphur in the soil are known to have significantly reduced concentrations of selenium in the diet due to the competitive absorption of sulphur over selenium [82]. Brazil nuts are particularly high in organic selenium content and can lead to over nutrition if consumed in substantial amounts [83]. Selenium can also be obtained from cereals and a variety of fruits and vegetables, with 30–40% of dietary intake found in meats, fish and poultry [84]. There are a number of markers of selenium concentrations in the body [85]. Urinary excretion of selenium should range between 15–50 μg/L and is a marker of intake status. Selenium status can also be measured within the blood serum where the reference range is between 70–150 ng/mL for adults and 45–90 ng/mL for newborns [16].

Selenium exerts its functions in the body in the form of selenocysteine (SeCys), the 21st amino acid in the body [86]. Selenoproteins often contain SeCys, the main selenoprotein families are the thioredoxin reductases (TRxR), glutathione peroxidases (GPx), and iodothyronine deiodinases (IDO) [87]. Both TRxR and GPx are antioxidants that protect the body from high levels of oxidative stress; whereas the IDO's are used to convert the inactive thyroid hormone, T4, to the biologically active form, T3 [88]. The thyroid is thus sensitive to selenium concentrations, and deficiency can result in an exacerbation of iodine deficiency [88]. As discussed subsequently, selenium deficiency during gestation has been associated with a number of negative outcomes, these include miscarriages, premature birth, low birth weight, and preeclampsia [36]. Consistently high levels of selenium intake can lead to selenosis: symptoms include gastrointestinal distress, hair loss, brittle fingernails and fatigue. Selenosis has also been shown to cause mild nerve damage and increase the risk of type-2 diabetes mellitus. The effects of overnutrition of selenium on offspring is unknown, however it may reduce the risk of maternal hyperthyroidism and lymphocytic thyroiditis [76].

4. Micronutrition in Gestational Complications

Poor micronutrition is often concomitant with increased incidence of gestational disorders such as GDM, PE, IUGR, and preterm pregnancies [10,11,16]. The literature surrounding micronutrition is also very complex, highlighting interactions that occur between various elements in physiological systems, and is limited with regards to heavy metals that are not classified as essential micronutrients.

4.1. Gestational Diabetes Mellitus

Gestational diabetes mellitus is a severe complication of pregnancy with an increasing prevalence, doubling incidence over an 8-year period [89,90]. The syndrome results from an impaired capacity of maternal beta cells to adapt to decreased insulin sensitivity that occurs during gestation, impairing glucose tolerance during pregnancy. The subsequent increased glucose levels that accompany GDM can further impair the development of the placenta and fetal growth [91]. In addition, maternal metabolic effects of GDM increase the chance of weight issues and poor pancreatic function. The effects on the foetus include increased adiposity and fetal hyperinsulinemia [92]. Poorly managed cases of GDM have been shown to result in increased cases of hypoglycaemia, primary caesarean deliveries, and large for gestational age offspring [93]. Although GDM can also cause IUGR, it is more likely to result in macrosomic foetuses [91].

Low levels of circulating potassium have been associated with impaired glucose tolerance due to the reduced ability for the pancreas to secret insulin [92]. Low selenium and chromium intake have also been associated with GDM [94]. Low serum concentrations and urinary excretion of zinc have been shown to be associated with diabetes [95] and zinc efficiency is also known to reduce growth factor signalling, particularly the insulin-like growth factor axis [96,97]. A review by Zhang, C. and Rawal, S. (2017) systematically evaluated the effects of iron intake, and iron status in GDM suggesting that a potential link between greater iron stores or status during gestation and an increased risk of GDM [98].

4.2. Pre-eclampsia

Occurring in approximately 3–5% of pregnancies, PE is associated with over 60,000 maternal deaths a year and increases perinatal mortality 5-fold [99]. Characterised by maternal endothelial cell dysfunction, resulting in symptoms that include maternal hypertension and proteinuria in late gestation; there is no current early means of detection for PE. Believed to originate from abnormal implantation and vascular development of the placenta, resulting in placental dysfunction, the initial cause of PE is poor uterine and placental perfusion, which can lead to hypoxic conditions and increased oxidative stress [100]. In some cases, the condition may progress to eclampsia, leading to seizures, coma, and ultimately death [101].

Hypertension exhibited with PE is linked to the sodium:potassium ratio. Blood pressure is correlated directly with sodium intake and inversely with potassium; however, potassium intake has not been associated with hypertensive disorders in pregnancy [102]. A systematic review of 13 studies on calcium supplementation during pregnancy found that with supplementation of 1 g/day, the average risk of PE was reduced by 55%, whilst gestational hypertensive disorders were reduced by 35% [103]. Due to magnesium deficiency being concomitant to calcium and potassium levels, it has been linked to PE. Magnesium levels in women with PE have been shown to be significantly reduced when compared to normal pregnant controls [46,104]. The decreased function of antioxidants that is accompanied with selenium and zinc deficiency has led to them being associated with preeclampsia, known to be correlated with high levels of oxidative stress [105].

4.3. Intrauterine Growth Restriction

Fetal growth restriction or IUGR occurs when the foetus fails to reach its expected growth potential at the appropriate gestational age. Associated with increased perinatal morbidity and mortality, IUGR is responsible for 30% of stillbirths, and increased incidence of premature births [106]. While IUGR babies may be born small for gestational age (SGA), IUGR babies are more likely to show signs of placental disease and have worse perinatal outcomes than SGA babies [107]. IUGR is mostly caused by the placenta through either poor placental function and/or insufficiency and a failure to adapt to improve fetal growth [108–110], this is known to be associated with an increase in diseases throughout life [111].

Reduced uterine blood flow may occur due to maternal hypotension or renal disease, which can lead to a reduced nutrient transport to the foetus which can cause IUGR [112,113]. Studies suggest that lower maternal manganese levels are associated with IUGR and an increased incidence of lower birth weight [114], whilst iron over nutrition has been linked to an increased possibility for SGA babies [16]. During pregnancy, a poor intake of zinc is teratogenic, causing IUGR and structural abnormalities [30,115]. Iodine deficiency is associated with a number of negative outcomes. Areas deficient in iodine see an increase in both birthweight and head circumference in offspring [116]. Low selenium intake has also been associated with IUGR, and recurrent miscarriage [32].

4.4. Preterm Birth

It's estimated 1:10 babies are born prematurely with approximately one million children dying each year due to complications associated with preterm birth. Factors such as maternal stress and inflammation have been associated, however literature suggests that placental ischemia or other forms of placental dysfunction are more likely to contribute to preterm birth [117]. There are higher rates of disability in children and increased risk of disease susceptibility throughout life with preterm births, with the chances increased the earlier a child is born [118,119].

Pre-term delivery was shown to be reduced in women supplemented with calcium. A WHO randomised control trial of >8000 women with <600 mg/day calcium intake showed that those with calcium supplementation had statistically lower incidence of pre-term birth than the placebo group (2.6% supplemented vs. 3.2% placebo) [120]. Low magnesium levels have also been correlated with increased incidence of pre-term birth and low birth weight in offspring in humans [45]. Iron deficiency has been associated with poor growth development, premature birth, and impairment of cognitive skills and neurodevelopment [16]. Women with low haemoglobin levels have been found to have double the risk of premature delivery and low birthweight in offspring [121,122]. Two studies have correlated low selenium concentrations in maternal and cord blood to pre-term birth, with evidence suggesting that adequate maternal selenium may protect against pre-term deliveries [123,124].

5. Profiling Micronutrients in Disease

The complexities surrounding micronutrition during pregnancy are profound. As previously stated, over and under nutrition of various elements can be correlated to diverse outcomes. Therefore, measuring a small number of variables in isolation may not be able to give an accurate representation of disease or be able to monitor disease progression. By measuring the pattern of many trace elements, various disease conditions may be better characterised and therefore treated. Early work using elemental metabolomics for Alzheimer's disease, Parkinson's, type 2 diabetes, and cancer has yielded promising results for both characterisation and understanding of disease.

Elemental Metabolomics

Elemental metabolomics (also known as ionomics), is a technique which involves the simultaneous quantification and characterisation of many chemical elements with high-throughput elemental analysis technologies and their integration with bioinformatics tools [125]. The concepts behind elemental metabolomics were established in the early 1940s, introducing terms like "metabolic patterns", "individual metabolic patterns", and "hypothetical average individual". It is only with recent advances in sensitivity, throughput, instrumentation, cheminformatics, and bioinformatics that determining the detailed metabolic pattern of an individual has become feasible [126]. This allows the establishment of "elemental signature which may prove to be powerful diagnostic aids.

The majority of techniques used in elemental analysis include inductively coupled plasma mass spectrometry (ICP-MS), inductively coupled plasma optical emission spectroscopy (ICP-OES), and X-ray fluorescence [127]. Among them, ICP-MS is the most frequently used approach, which is capable of detecting metals as low as parts per trillion. Compared to other methodologies, ICP-MS allows for smaller sample size owing to its greater sensitivity and has the ability to detect different isotopes of the same element (Figure 1) Currently, ICP-MS has been successfully used for large scale elemental studies in yeast, plants and mammals [128,129]. These investigations illustrate the power of metabolomics to identify new aspects of trace element metabolism and homeostasis, and how such information can be used to develop hypotheses regarding the functions of previously uncharacterised diseases [130,131].

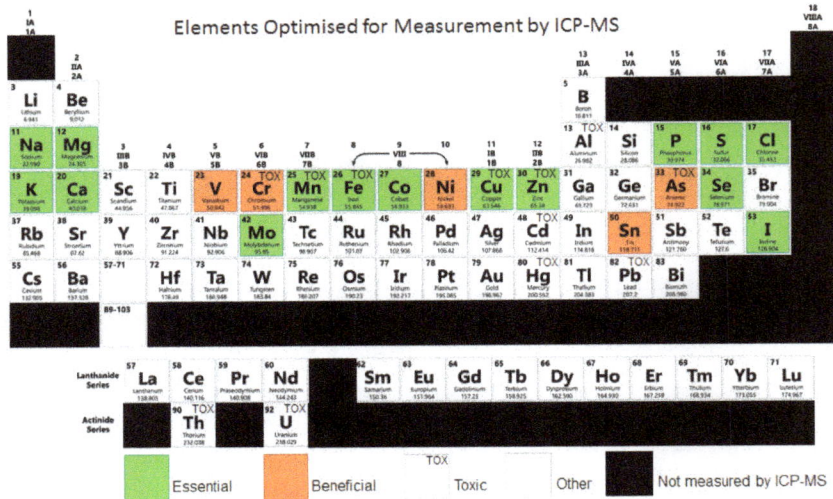

Figure 1. Elements measurable by ICP-MS, image adapted from Zhang, P. et al., (2017) [126]. Classified into essential, beneficial, others without a clearly defined function, and toxic elements. Essential and beneficial elements comprise major structural components (Ca, P, S); components of hormones or enzymes (Co, Cr, Cu, Fe, I, Mn, Mo, Ni, Se, Sn, V, Zn); responsible for maintenance of ionic equilibria, activation, or signalling (Ca, K, Mg, Na).

ICP-MS has been used for the quantification of elements in a variety of different human diseases, but the pattern of elements in disease states are far less well categorised. Even so, the limited work that has been conducted in the medical field has yielded promising results for various conditions such as Alzheimer's disease, Parkinson's, type 2 diabetes, and cancer. Little work has been conducted on the determination of elemental metabolomic profiles during gestation. Once established, elemental metabolomic profiles could better characterise various biological conditions and pathologies, providing novel treatment options. For example, recently it has been shown that metabolomics can identify genes and gene networks that directly control the metabolome [131]. In addition, this technique may provide a powerful tool for investigating more complex networks in gestation that control developmental and physiological processes that influence the metabolome indirectly.

With the accelerated development of elemental metabolomics, advanced strategies have been developed for systematic analysis of chemical elements. A recent study identified a distinctive pattern of serum elements during the progression of Alzheimer's disease. With the metabolomic analysis of elemental ratios, this study was able to differentiate with 90% accuracy between diseased and healthy individuals. Essential elements such as manganese, selenium, zinc and iron were shown to increase initially with early onset of Alzheimer's then decrease with the development of mild cognitive impairment and ultimately true Alzheimer's disease [12].

In another study, trace elements in plasma were analysed for 238 diagnosed Parkinson's patients and 302 controls. Their findings indicated that lower plasma selenium and iron concentrations may reduce the risk of developing the disease, whereas lower plasma zinc was associated with an increased risk factor. They also used a model to then predict patient disease status based on several trace elements, also defining other features such as sex and age, highlighting possibilities for future computational strategies to improve elemental metabolomic studies [13].

Sun et al., analysed the fasting elemental concentrations of 976 middle-aged Chinese men and women to determine associations of ion modules and networks with obesity, metabolic syndrome, and type 2 diabetes mellitus (T2D). They found that copper and phosphorus were always ranked as the first two specific ion networks in people with health complications, whilst specific elemental patterns were also observed for each of the conditions [132]. Another study noted that increased urinary nickel concentrations were associated with an increased incidence of T2D in 2115 Chinese aged 55–76 years old [14].

Golasik et al., investigated the relationship between elemental status and cancer risk to support diagnosis. Disturbance in the homeostasis of metals is among one of many factors that can cause cancer malignancy. Through analysing both essential elements (calcium, magnesium, zinc, manganese, copper, iron etc.) and toxic elements (cadmium and lead) in hair and nail samples of patients with laryngeal cancer, they noted that most of the essential elements were significantly reduced in cancer patients, whilst toxic elements increased. Using a variety of bioinformatic techniques they were also able to determine classifiers for prediction of cancer probability, which may be useful for estimating risk, and early screening of cancer [15].

Elemental studies have also been used to examine metal concentrations in saliva and blood of periodontal disease patients. Using cluster analysis of metals in the classifications of samples, the resulting clusters suggested the elemental profiles of those with periodontal disease are different from controls. These researchers concluded that this may become a basis for future diagnostic and prognostic tools for periodontal disease [133].

6. Conclusions

Gestational complications such as GDM, PE, IUGR, and preterm birth can have lifelong consequences for the health of the mother and child. However, pregnancy disorders such as these are poorly understood despite extensive research. Little work has been conducted on the determination of elemental metabolomic profiles during gestation and how this might be influenced by maternal nutrition. Once established, elemental metabolomic profiles could better characterise various biological conditions and pathologies, providing novel treatment options. Currently, we only know how a select few micronutrients affect pregnancy outcomes [25], even though many additional micronutrients are likely to be essential to human development.

Development of elemental metabolomic technology for generating a micronutrient "signature" or "fingerprint" as a predictive biomarker of pregnancy complications could provide vital information on relationships between specific micronutrients and pregnancy complications. Many key proteins in the body require specific micronutrients to function, therefore screening to identify novel and subtle micronutrient changes could highlight associated proteins that may affected and underpinning the pathophysiology of these complications. This would open up the way for simple interventions and therapies which could prove to be of immense benefit to both mother and baby.

Author Contributions: Conceptualization, D.R.M., A.V.P.; Resources, A.V.P.; Writing—Original Draft Preparation, D.R.M., J.J.F.; Writing—Review & Editing, J.J.F., A.V.P.; Supervision, A.V.P.

Funding: The research of D.R.M. and J.J.F. is supported by the Griffith University Postgraduate research scholarship (GUPRS).

Conflicts of Interest: The authors declare no conflict of interest.

References

1. Mertz, W. The essential trace elements. *Science* **1981**, *213*, 1332–1338. [CrossRef]
2. Australian Bureau of Statistics: A.B.O. National Health Survey: First Results, 2014-15. Cat. no. 4364.0. 55.001. Available online: http://www.abs.gov.au/AUSSTATS/abs@.nsf/DetailsPage/4364.0.55.0012014-15?OpenDocument (accessed on 18 October 2015).
3. Abu-Saad, K.; Fraser, D. Maternal nutrition and birth outcomes. *Epidemiol. Rev.* **2010**, *32*, 5–25. [CrossRef] [PubMed]
4. Blumfield, M.L.; Hure, A.J.; Macdonald-Wicks, L.; Smith, R.; Collins, C.E. A systematic review and meta-analysis of micronutrient intakes during pregnancy in developed countries. *Nutr. Rev.* **2013**, *71*, 118–132. [CrossRef] [PubMed]

5. Darnton-Hill, I.; Mkparu, U.C. Micronutrients in pregnancy in low- and middle-income countries. *Nutrients* **2015**, *7*, 1744–1768. [CrossRef] [PubMed]

6. WHO/FAO. *Vitamin and Mineral Requirements in Human Nutrition*, 2nd ed.; World Health Organization and Food and Agriculture Organization of the United Nations: Geneva, Switzerland, 2004.

7. Ahmed, T.; Hossain, M.; Sanin, K.I. Global burden of maternal and child undernutrition and micronutrient deficiencies. *Ann. Nutr. Metab.* **2012**, *61*, 8–17. [CrossRef] [PubMed]

8. New Zealand Ministry of Health. Nutrient Reference Values for Australia and New Zealand. Available online: https://www.health.govt.nz/publication/nutrient-reference-values-australia-and-new-zealand (accessed on 21 October 2015).

9. Vanderlelie, J.; Scott, R.; Shibl, R.; Lewkowicz, J.; Perkins, A.; Scuffham, P.A. First trimester multivitamin/mineral use is associated with reduced risk of pre-eclampsia among overweight and obese women. *Matern. Child Nutr.* **2016**, *12*, 339–348. [CrossRef] [PubMed]

10. Gernand, A.D.; Schulze, K.J.; Stewart, C.P.; West, K.P., Jr.; Christian, P. Micronutrient deficiencies in pregnancy worldwide: Health effects and prevention. *Nat. Rev. Endocrinol.* **2016**, *12*, 274–289. [CrossRef] [PubMed]

11. Cheong, J.N.; Wlodek, M.E.; Moritz, K.M.; Cuffe, J.S. Programming of maternal and offspring disease: Impact of growth restriction, fetal sex and transmission across generations. *J. Physiol.* **2016**, *594*, 4727–4740. [CrossRef]

12. Paglia, G.; Miedico, O.; Cristofano, A.; Vitale, M.; Angiolillo, A.; Chiaravalle, A.E.; Corso, G.; Di Costanzo, A. Distinctive pattern of serum elements during the progression of Alzheimer's disease. *Sci. Rep.* **2016**, *6*, 22769. [CrossRef]

13. Zhao, H.-W.; Lin, J.; Wang, X.-B.; Cheng, X.; Wang, J.-Y.; Hu, B.-L.; Zhang, Y.; Zhang, X.; Zhu, J.-H. Assessing plasma levels of selenium, copper, iron and zinc in patients of Parkinson's disease. *PLoS ONE* **2013**, *8*, e83060. [CrossRef]

14. Liu, G.; Sun, L.; Pan, A.; Zhu, M.; Li, Z.; Wang, Z.; Liu, X.; Ye, X.; Li, H.; Zheng, H. Nickel exposure is associated with the prevalence of type 2 diabetes in Chinese adults. *Int. J. Epidemiol.* **2014**, *44*, 240–248. [CrossRef] [PubMed]

15. Golasik, M.; Jawień, W.; Przybyłowicz, A.; Szyfter, W.; Herman, M.; Golusiński, W.; Florek, E.; Piekoszewski, W. Classification models based on the level of metals in hair and nails of laryngeal cancer patients: Diagnosis support or rather speculation? *Metallomics* **2015**, *7*, 455–465. [CrossRef] [PubMed]

16. Gluckman, P.; Hanson, M.; Seng, C.Y.; Bardsley, A. *Nutrition and Lifestyle for Pregnancy and Breastfeeding*; Oxford University Press: Oxford, UK, 2014.

17. Fall, C.H.; Fisher, D.J.; Osmond, C.; Margetts, B.M. Multiple micronutrient supplementation during pregnancy in low-income countries: A meta-analysis of effects on birth size and length of gestation. *Food Nutr. Bull.* **2009**, *30*, S533–S546. [CrossRef] [PubMed]

18. Gaccioli, F.; Lager, S. Placental nutrient transport and intrauterine growth restriction. *Front. Physiol.* **2016**, *7*, 40. [CrossRef] [PubMed]

19. Antony, A.C. Folate receptors. *Annu.Rev. Nutr.* **1996**, *16*, 501–521. [CrossRef] [PubMed]

20. Solanky, N.; Jimenez, A.R.; D'Souza, S.; Sibley, C.; Glazier, J. Expression of folate transporters in human placenta and implications for homocysteine metabolism. *Placenta* **2010**, *31*, 134–143. [CrossRef] [PubMed]

21. Barker, D.J.; Osmond, C. Infant mortality, childhood nutrition, and ischaemic heart disease in England and Wales. *Lancet* **1986**, *327*, 1077–1081. [CrossRef]

22. Thornburg, K.L.; Shannon, J.; Thuillier, P.; Turker, M.S. In utero life and epigenetic predisposition for disease. *Adv. Genet.* **2010**, *71*, 57.

23. Roseboom, T.J.; Van Der Meulen, J.H.; Ravelli, A.C.; Osmond, C.; Barker, D.J.; Bleker, O.P. Effects of prenatal exposure to the Dutch famine on adult disease in later life: An overview. *Mol. Cell. Endocrinol.* **2001**, *185*, 93–98. [CrossRef]

24. Grieger, J.A.; Clifton, V.L. A review of the impact of dietary intakes in human pregnancy on infant birthweight. *Nutrients* **2014**, *7*, 153–178. [CrossRef]

25. Lewicka, I.; Kocyłowski, R.; Grzesiak, M.; Gaj, Z.; Oszukowski, P.; Suliburska, J. Selected trace elements concentrations in pregnancy and their possible role—Literature review. *Ginekol. Pol.* **2017**, *88*, 509–514. [CrossRef] [PubMed]

26. Burtis, C.A.; Ashwood, E.R.; Bruns, D.E. *Tietz Textbook of Clinical Chemistry and Molecular Diagnostics*; Elsevier Saunders: Philadelphia, PA, USA, 2006.

27. Matsunami, K.; Imai, A.; Tamaya, T. Hypokalemia in a pregnant woman with long-term heavy cola consumption. *Int. J. Gynecol. Obstet.* **1994**, *44*, 283–284. [CrossRef]

28. Appel, C.C.; Myles, T.D. Caffeine-induced hypokalemic paralysis in pregnancy. *Obstet. Gynecol.* **2001**, *97*, 805–807. [PubMed]

29. Khaw, K.; Barrett-Connor, E. The association between blood pressure, age, and dietary sodium and potassium: A population study. *Circulation* **1988**, *77*, 53–61. [CrossRef] [PubMed]

30. Hofstee, P.; McKeating, D.R.; Perkins, A.V.; Cuffe, J.S. Placental adaptations to micronutrient dysregulation in the programming of chronic disease. *Clin. Exp. Pharmacol. Physiol.* **2018**, *45*, 871–884. [CrossRef] [PubMed]

31. Wolak, T.; Shoham-Vardi, I.; Sergienko, R.; Sheiner, E. High potassium level during pregnancy is associated with future cardiovascular morbidity. *J. Matern. Fetal Neonatal Med.* **2016**, *29*, 1021–1024. [CrossRef]

32. Farinde, A. Lab Values, Normal Adult: Laboratory Reference Ranges in Healthy Adults. Available online: https://emedicine.medscape.com/article/2172316-overview (accessed on 16 April 2018).

33. FSANZ. *The 23rd Australian Total Diet Study*; Food Standards Australia New Zealand: Barton, ACT, Australia, 2011.

34. Jantzen, C.; Jørgensen, H.L.; Duus, B.R.; Sporring, S.L.; Lauritzen, J.B. Chromium and cobalt ion concentrations in blood and serum following various types of metal-on-metal hip arthroplasties: A literature overview. *Acta Orthop.* **2013**, *84*, 229–236. [CrossRef]

35. Galinier, A.; Périquet, B.; Lambert, W.; Garcia, J.; Assouline, C.; Rolland, M.; Thouvenot, J.-P. Reference range for micronutrients and nutritional marker proteins in cord blood of neonates appropriated for gestational ages. *Early Human Dev.* **2005**, *81*, 583–593. [CrossRef]

36. Mariath, A.B.; Bergamaschi, D.P.; Rondó, P.H.; Ana, C.A.T.; de Fragas Hinnig, P.; Abbade, J.F.; Diniz, S.G. The possible role of selenium status in adverse pregnancy outcomes. *Br. J. Nutr.* **2011**, *105*, 1418–1428. [CrossRef]

37. Brown, E.M. *Vitamin D and the Calcium-Sensing Receptor. Vitamin D*, 3rd ed.; Elsevier: New York, NY, USA, 2011; pp. 425–456.

38. Brini, M.; Ottolini, D.; Calì, T.; Carafoli, E. Calcium in health and disease. In *Interrelations between Essential Metal Ions and Human Diseases*; Sigel, A., Sigel, H., Sigel, R., Eds.; Springer: Berlin, Germany, 2013; pp. 81–137.

39. Jorde, R.; Sundsfjord, J.; Haug, E.; Bønaa, K.H. Relation between low calcium intake, parathyroid hormone, and blood pressure. *Hypertension* **2000**, *35*, 1154–1159. [CrossRef]

40. Lumbers, E.R.; Pringle, K.G. Roles of the circulating renin-angiotensin-aldosterone system in human pregnancy. *Am. J. Physiol. Regul. Integr. Comp. Physiol.* **2013**, *306*, R91–R101. [CrossRef] [PubMed]

41. Imdad, A.; Bhutta, Z.A. Effects of calcium supplementation during pregnancy on maternal, fetal and birth outcomes. *Paediatr. Perinat. Epidemiol.* **2012**, *26*, 138–152. [CrossRef] [PubMed]

42. Fatemi, S.; Ryzen, E.; Flores, J.; Endres, D.B.; Rude, R.K. Effect of experimental human magnesium depletion on parathyroid hormone secretion and 1,25-dihydroxyvitamin D metabolism. *J. Clin. Endocrinol. Metab.* **1991**, *73*, 1067–1072. [CrossRef] [PubMed]

43. Arnaud, M.J. Update on the assessment of magnesium status. *Br. J. Nutr.* **2008**, *99*, S24–S36. [CrossRef] [PubMed]

44. Rude, R.K. Magnesium deficiency: A cause of heterogenous disease in humans. *J. Bone Miner. Res.* **1998**, *13*, 749–758. [CrossRef] [PubMed]

45. Spencer, B.; Vanderlelie, J.; Perkins, A. Essentiality of trace element micronutrition in human pregnancy: A systematic review. *J. Pregnancy Child Health* **2015**, *2*, 2. [CrossRef]

46. Williams, M.; Todd, G.; Roney, N.; Crawford, J.; Coles, C.; McClure, P.; Garey, J.; Zaccaria, K.; Citra, M. *Toxicological Profile for Manganese*; Agency for Toxic Substances and Disease Registry: Atlanta, GA, USA, 2012.

47. Fitsanakis, V.A.; Zhang, N.; Garcia, S.; Aschner, M. Manganese (Mn) and iron (Fe): Interdependency of transport and regulation. *Neurotox. Res.* **2010**, *18*, 124–131. [CrossRef]

48. Greger, J. Dietary standards for manganese: Overlap between nutritional and toxicological studies. *J. Nutr.* **1998**, *128*, 368S–371S. [CrossRef]

49. Freeland-Graves, J.H.; Lin, P.-H. Plasma uptake of manganese as affected by oral loads of manganese, calcium, milk, phosphorus, copper, and zinc. *J. Am. Coll. Nutr.* **1991**, *10*, 38–43. [CrossRef]

50. Law, N.A.; Caudle, M.T.; Pecoraro, V.L. Manganese redox enzymes and model systems: Properties, structures, and reactivity. *Adv. Inorg. Chem.* **1998**, *46*, 305–440.

51. Davis, C.D.; Greger, J. Longitudinal changes of manganese-dependent superoxide dismutase and other indexes of manganese and iron status in women. *Am. J. Clin. Nutr.* **1992**, *55*, 747–752. [CrossRef]

52. Friedman, B.; Freeland-Graves, J.H.; Bales, C.W.; Behmardi, F.; Shorey-Kutschke, R.L.; Willis, R.A.; Crosby, J.B.; Trickett, P.C.; Houston, S.D. Manganese balance and clinical observations in young men fed a manganese-deficient diet. *J. Nutr.* **1987**, *117*, 133–143. [CrossRef] [PubMed]

53. Tholin, K.; Sandström, B.; Palm, R.; Hallmans, G. Changes in blood manganese levels during pregnancy in iron supplemented and non supplemented women. *J. Trace Elem. Med. Biol.* **1995**, *9*, 13–17. [CrossRef]

54. Spencer, A. Whole blood manganese levels in pregnancy and the neonate. *Nutrition* **1999**, *15*, 731–734. [CrossRef]

55. Henn, B.C.; Bellinger, D.C.; Hopkins, M.R.; Coull, B.A.; Ettinger, A.S.; Jim, R.; Hatley, E.; Christiani, D.C.; Wright, R.O. Maternal and cord blood manganese concentrations and early childhood neurodevelopment among residents near a mining-impacted superfund site. *Environ. Health Perspect.* **2017**, *125*. [CrossRef]

56. Institute of Medicine Dietary. *Vitamin A, Vitamin K, Arsenic, Boron, Chromium, Copper, Iodine, Iron, Manganese, Molybdenum, Nickel, Silicon, Vanadium, and Zinc*; Institute of Medicine National Academy Press: Washington, WA, USA, 2001.

57. Hulten, L.; Gramatkovski, E.; Gleerup, A.; Hallberg, L. Iron absorption from the whole diet. Relation to meal composition, iron requirements and iron stores. *Eur. J. Clin. Nutr.* **1995**, *49*, 794–808. [PubMed]

58. Hider, R.C.; Kong, X. Iron: Effect of overload and deficiency. *Met. Ions Life Sci.* **2013**, *13*, 229–294. [PubMed]

59. Henderson, B.; Kühn, L. Interaction between iron-regulatory proteins and their RNA target sequences, iron-responsive elements. *Prog. Mol. Subcell. Biol.* **1997**, *18*, 17–139.

60. Koulaouzidis, A.; Said, E.; Cottier, R.; Saeed, A.A. Soluble transferrin receptors and iron deficiency, a step beyond ferritin. A systematic review. *J. Gastrointest. Liver Dis.* **2009**, *18*, 345–352.

61. Dandona, P.; Hussain, M.; Varghese, Z.; Politis, D.; Flynn, D.; Hoffbrand, A. Insulin resistance and iron overload. *Ann. Clin. Biochem.* **1983**, *20*, 77–79. [CrossRef] [PubMed]

62. Peña, M.M.; Lee, J.; Thiele, D.J. A delicate balance: Homeostatic control of copper uptake and distribution. *J. Nutr.* **1999**, *129*, 1251–1260. [CrossRef] [PubMed]

63. McKeown, N.M. Whole grain intake and insulin sensitivity: Evidence from observational studies. *Nutr. Rev.* **2004**, *62*, 286. [PubMed]

64. Trumbo, P.; Schlicker, S.; Yates, A.A.; Poos, M. Dietary reference intakes for energy, carbohydrate, fiber, fat, fatty acids, cholesterol, protein and amino acids. *J. Am. Diet. Assoc.* **2002**, *102*, 1621–1630. [CrossRef]

65. Drehmer, M.; Camey, S.A.; Nunes, M.A.; Duncan, B.B.; Lacerda, M.; Pinheiro, A.P.; Schmidt, M.I. Fibre intake and evolution of BMI: From pre-pregnancy to postpartum. *Public Health Nutr.* **2013**, *16*, 1403–1413. [CrossRef] [PubMed]

66. Klevay, L.M. Is the Western diet adequate in copper? *J. Trace Elem. Med. Biol.* **2011**, *25*, 204–212. [CrossRef]

67. Al-Rashid, R.A.; Spangler, J. Neonatal copper deficiency. *N. Engl. J. Med.* **1971**, *285*, 841–843. [CrossRef]

68. Prasad, A.S. Impact of the discovery of human zinc deficiency on health. *J. Trace Elem. Med. Biol.* **2014**, *28*, 357–363. [CrossRef]

69. Andreini, C.; Banci, L.; Bertini, I.; Rosato, A. Counting the zinc-proteins encoded in the human genome. *J. Proteome Res.* **2006**, *5*, 196–201. [CrossRef]

70. Foster, M.; Herulah, U.N.; Prasad, A.; Petocz, P.; Samman, S. Zinc status of vegetarians during pregnancy: A systematic review of observational studies and meta-analysis of zinc intake. *Nutrients* **2015**, *7*, 4512–4525. [CrossRef]

71. O'Dell, B.L. Role of zinc in plasma membrane function. *J. Nutr.* **2000**, *130*, 1432S–1436S. [CrossRef]

72. Mossad, S.B.; Macknin, M.L.; Mendendorp, S.V.; Mason, P. Zinc gluconate lozenges for treating the common cold: A randomized, double-blind, placebo-controlled study. *Ann. Intern. Med.* **1996**, *125*, 81–88. [CrossRef] [PubMed]

73. Andersson, M.; De Benoist, B.; Darnton-Hill, I.; Delange, F.M.; Organization, W.H.; UNICEF. *Iodine Deficiency in Europe: A Continuing Public Health Problem*; WHO: Geneva, Switzerland, 2007.

74. Hetzel, B.S. Iodine and neuropsychological development. *J. Nutr.* **2000**, *130*, 493S–495S. [CrossRef] [PubMed]

75. Vejbjerg, P.; Knudsen, N.; Perrild, H.; Laurberg, P.; Andersen, S.; Rasmussen, L.B.; Ovesen, L.; Jørgensen, T. Estimation of iodine intake from various urinary iodine measurements in population studies. *Thyroid* **2009**, *19*, 1281–1286. [CrossRef] [PubMed]

76. Richard, K.; Holland, O.; Landers, K.; Vanderlelie, J.J.; Hofstee, P.; Cuffe, J.S.; Perkins, A.V. Review: Effects of maternal micronutrient supplementation on placental function. *Placenta* **2017**, *54*, 38–44. [CrossRef] [PubMed]

77. Vermiglio, F.; Lo Presti, V.P.; Moleti, M.; Sidoti, M.; Tortorella, G.; Scaffidi, G.; Castagna, M.G.; Mattina, F.; Violi, M.A.; Crisa, A.; et al. Attention deficit and hyperactivity disorders in the offspring of mothers exposed to mild-moderate iodine deficiency: A possible novel iodine deficiency disorder in developed countries. *J. Clin. Endocrinol. Metab.* **2004**, *89*, 6054–6060. [CrossRef] [PubMed]

78. Sang, Z.; Wei, W.; Zhao, N.; Zhang, G.; Chen, W.; Liu, H.; Shen, J.; Liu, J.; Yan, Y.; Zhang, W. Thyroid dysfunction during late gestation is associated with excessive iodine intake in pregnant women. *J. Clin. Endocrinol. Metab.* **2012**, *97*, E1363–E1369. [CrossRef]

79. Connelly, K.J.; Boston, B.A.; Pearce, E.N.; Sesser, D.; Snyder, D.; Braverman, L.E.; Pino, S.; LaFranchi, S.H. Congenital hypothyroidism caused by excess prenatal maternal iodine ingestion. *J. Pediatr.* **2012**, *161*, 760–762. [CrossRef] [PubMed]

80. Besser, J.M.; Canfield, T.J.; La Point, T.W. Bioaccumulation of organic and inorganic selenium in a laboratory food chain. *Environ. Toxicol. Chem.* **1993**, *12*, 57–72. [CrossRef]

81. Institute of Medicine, Food and Nutrition Board. *Dietary Reference Intakes: Vitamin C, Vitamin E, Selenium, and Carotenoids*; National Academy Press: Washington, WA, USA, 2000.

82. Liu, X.; Zhao, Z.; Duan, B.; Hu, C.; Zhao, X.; Guo, Z. Effect of applied sulphur on the uptake by wheat of selenium applied as selenite. *Plant Soil* **2015**, *386*, 35–45. [CrossRef]

83. Navarro-Alarcon, M.; Cabrera-Vique, C. Selenium in food and the human body: A review. *Sci. Total Environ.* **2008**, *400*, 115–141. [CrossRef]

84. Dumont, E.; De Pauw, L.; Vanhaecke, F.; Cornelis, R. Speciation of se in Bertholletia excelsa (Brazil nut): A hard nut to crack? *Food Chem.* **2006**, *95*, 684–692. [CrossRef]

85. Dumont, E.; Vanhaecke, F.; Cornelis, R. Selenium speciation from food source to metabolites: A critical review. *Anal. Bioanal. Chem.* **2006**, *385*, 1304–1323. [CrossRef] [PubMed]

86. Korotkov, K.V.; Novoselov, S.V.; Hatfield, D.L.; Gladyshev, V.N. Mammalian selenoprotein in which selenocysteine (Sec) incorporation is supported by a new form of Sec insertion sequence element. *Mol. Cell. Biol.* **2002**, *22*, 1402–1411. [CrossRef] [PubMed]

87. Papp, L.V.; Lu, J.; Holmgren, A.; Khanna, K.K. From selenium to selenoproteins: Synthesis, identity, and their role in human health. *Antioxid. Redox Signal.* **2007**, *9*, 775–806. [CrossRef] [PubMed]

88. Zimmermann, M.B.; Köhrle, J. The impact of iron and selenium deficiencies on iodine and thyroid metabolism: Biochemistry and relevance to public health. *Thyroid* **2002**, *12*, 867–878. [CrossRef] [PubMed]

89. Lawrence, J.M.; Contreras, R.; Chen, W.; Sacks, D.A. Trends in the prevalence of preexisting diabetes and gestational diabetes mellitus among a racially/ethnically diverse population of pregnant women, 1999–2005. *Diabetes Care* **2008**, *31*, 899–904. [CrossRef]

90. Dabelea, D.; Snell-Bergeon, J.K.; Hartsfield, C.L.; Bischoff, K.J.; Hamman, R.F.; McDuffie, R.S. Increasing prevalence of gestational diabetes mellitus (GDM) over time and by birth cohort: Kaiser permanente of Colorado GDM screening program. *Diabetes Care* **2005**, *28*, 579–584. [CrossRef]

91. Jameson, J.L.; De Groot, L.J. *Endocrinology: Adult and Pediatric*, 7th ed.; Elsevier Saunders: Philadelphia, PA, USA, 2015; pp. 788–804.

92. Chatterjee, R.; Yeh, H.-C.; Edelman, D.; Brancati, F. Potassium and risk of type 2 diabetes. *Expert Rev. Endocrinol. Metab.* **2011**, *6*, 665–672. [CrossRef]

93. Vambergue, A.; Fajardy, I. Consequences of gestational and pregestational diabetes on placental function and birth weight. *World J. Diabetes* **2011**, *2*, 196. [CrossRef]

94. Basaki, M.; Saeb, M.; Nazifi, S.; Shamsaei, H. Zinc, copper, iron, and chromium concentrations in young patients with type 2 diabetes mellitus. *Biol. Trace Elem. Res.* **2012**, *148*, 161–164. [CrossRef]

95. El-Yazigi, A.; Hannan, N.; Raines, D.A. Effect of diabetic state and related disorders on the urinary excretion of magnesium and zinc in patients. *Diabetes Research Edinb. Scotl.* **1993**, *22*, 67–75.

96. Jansen, J.; Rosenkranz, E.; Overbeck, S.; Warmuth, S.; Mocchegiani, E.; Giacconi, R.; Weiskirchen, R.; Karges, W.; Rink, L. Disturbed zinc homeostasis in diabetic patients by in vitro and in vivo analysis of insulinomimetic activity of zinc. *J. Nutr. Biochem.* **2012**, *23*, 1458–1466. [CrossRef] [PubMed]

97. MacDonald, R.S. The role of zinc in growth and cell proliferation. *J. Nutr.* **2000**, *130*, 1500S–1508S. [CrossRef]

98. Zhang, C.; Rawal, S. Dietary iron intake, iron status, and gestational diabetes. *Am. J. Clin. Nutr.* **2017**, *106*, 1672S–1680S. [CrossRef] [PubMed]

99. Roberts, J.M. Preeclampsia: What we know and what we do not know. *Semin. Perinatol.* **2000**, *24*, 24–28. [CrossRef]

100. McDonald, S.D.; Han, Z.; Walsh, M.W.; Gerstein, H.C.; Devereaux, P.J. Kidney disease after preeclampsia: A systematic review and meta-analysis. *Am. J. Kidney Dis.* **2010**, *55*, 1026–1039. [CrossRef]

101. Ghulmiyyah, L.; Sibai, B. Maternal mortality from preeclampsia/eclampsia. *Semin. Perinatol.* **2012**, *36*, 56–59. [CrossRef]

102. Morris, C.D.; Jacobson, S.-L.; Anand, R.; Ewell, M.G.; Hauth, J.C.; Curet, L.B.; Catalano, P.M.; Sibai, B.M.; Levine, R.J. Nutrient intake and hypertensive disorders of pregnancy: Evidence from a large prospective cohort. *Am. J. Obstet. Gynecol.* **2001**, *184*, 643–651. [CrossRef]

103. Hofmeyr, G.J.; Lawrie, T.A.; Atallah, A.N.; Duley, L. Calcium supplementation during pregnancy for preventing hypertensive disorders and related problems. *Cochrane Database Syst. Rev.* **2010**. [CrossRef]

104. Jain, S.; Sharma, P.; Kulshreshtha, S.; Mohan, G.; Singh, S. The role of calcium, magnesium, and zinc in pre-eclampsia. *Biol. Trace Elem. Res.* **2010**, *133*, 162–170. [CrossRef]

105. Mistry, H.D.; Pipkin, F.B.; Redman, C.W.; Poston, L. Selenium in reproductive health. *Am. J. Obstet. Gynecol.* **2012**, *206*, 21–30. [CrossRef] [PubMed]

106. Ergaz, Z.; Avgil, M.; Ornoy, A. Intrauterine growth restriction—Etiology and consequences: What do we know about the human situation and experimental animal models? *Reprod. Toxicol.* **2005**, *20*, 301–322. [CrossRef] [PubMed]

107. Herrera, E.A.; Alegría, R.; Farias, M.; Díaz-López, F.; Hernández, C.; Uauy, R.; Regnault, T.R.; Casanello, P.; Krause, B.J. Assessment of in vivo fetal growth and placental vascular function in a novel intrauterine growth restriction model of progressive uterine artery occlusion in guinea pigs. *J. Physiol.* **2016**, *594*, 1553–1561. [CrossRef] [PubMed]

108. Nardozza, L.M.M.; Araujo Júnior, E.; Barbosa, M.M.; Caetano, A.C.R.; Lee, D.J.R.; Moron, A.F. Fetal growth restriction: Current knowledge to the general Obs/Gyn. *Arch. Gynecol. Obstet.* **2012**, *286*, 1–13. [CrossRef]

109. Figueras, F.; Gratacos, E. Stage-based approach to the management of fetal growth restriction. *Prenat. Diagn.* **2014**, *34*, 655–659. [CrossRef]

110. Henriksen, T.; Clausen, T. The fetal origins hypothesis: Placental insufficiency and inheritance versus maternal malnutrition in well-nourished populations. *Acta Obstet. Gynecol. Scand.* **2002**, *81*, 112–114. [CrossRef] [PubMed]

111. Coan, P.M.; Vaughan, O.R.; Sekita, Y.; Finn, S.L.; Burton, G.J.; Constancia, M.; Fowden, A.L. Adaptations in placental phenotype support fetal growth during undernutrition of pregnant mice. *J. Physiol.* **2010**, *588*, 527–538. [CrossRef]

112. Sandovici, I.; Hoelle, K.; Angiolini, E.; Constância, M. Placental adaptations to the maternal–fetal environment: Implications for fetal growth and developmental programming. *Reprod. Biomed. Online* **2012**, *25*, 68–89. [CrossRef]

113. Moore, K.L.; Persaud, T.V.N.; Torchia, M. *The developing human: Clinically Oriented Embryology*, 10th ed.; Elsevier: Philadelphia, PA, USA, 2015.

114. Wood, R.J. Manganese and birth outcome. *Nutr. Rev.* **2009**, *67*, 416–420. [CrossRef]

115. Wang, H.; Hu, Y.-F.; Hao, J.-H.; Chen, Y.-H.; Su, P.-Y.; Wang, Y.; Yu, Z.; Fu, L.; Xu, Y.-Y.; Zhang, C. Maternal zinc deficiency during pregnancy elevates the risks of fetal growth restriction: A population-based birth cohort study. *Sci. Rep.* **2015**, *5*, 11262. [CrossRef]

116. Cao, X.-Y.; Jiang, X.-M.; Dou, Z.-H.; Rakeman, M.A.; Zhang, M.-L.; O'Donnell, K.; Ma, T.; Amette, K.; DeLong, N.; DeLong, G.R. Timing of vulnerability of the brain to iodine deficiency in endemic cretinism. *N. Engl. J. Med.* **1994**, *331*, 1739–1744. [CrossRef] [PubMed]

117. Goldenberg, R.L.; Culhane, J.F.; Iams, J.D.; Romero, R. Epidemiology and causes of preterm birth. *Lancet* **2008**, *371*, 75–84. [CrossRef]

118. Schieve, L.A.; Tian, L.H.; Rankin, K.; Kogan, M.D.; Yeargin-Allsopp, M.; Visser, S.; Rosenberg, D. Population impact of preterm birth and low birth weight on developmental disabilities in US children. *Ann. Epidemiol.* **2016**, *26*, 267–274. [CrossRef] [PubMed]

119. Crump, C.; Sundquist, K.; Sundquist, J. Adult outcomes of preterm birth. *Prev. Med.* **2016**, *91*, 400–401. [CrossRef]

120. Villar, J.; Abdel-Aleem, H.; Merialdi, M.; Mathai, M.; Ali, M.M.; Zavaleta, N.; Purwar, M.; Hofmeyr, J.; Campódonico, L.; Landoulsi, S. World Health Organization randomized trial of calcium supplementation among low calcium intake pregnant women. *Am. J. Obstet. Gynecol.* **2006**, *194*, 639–649. [CrossRef] [PubMed]

121. Lieberman, E.; Ryan, K.J.; Monson, R.R.; Schoenbaum, S.C. Association of maternal hematocrit with premature labor. *Am. J. Obstet. Gynecol.* **1988**, *159*, 107–114. [CrossRef]

122. Scholl, T.O.; Hediger, M.L.; Fischer, R.L.; Shearer, J.W. Anemia vs iron deficiency: Increased risk of preterm delivery in a prospective study. *Am. J. Clin. Nutr.* **1992**, *55*, 985–988. [CrossRef] [PubMed]

123. Dobrzynski, W.; Szymanski, W.; Zachara, B.A.; Trafikowska, U.; Trafikowska, A.; Pilecki, A. Decreased selenium concentration in maternal and cord blood in preterm compared with term delivery. *Analyst* **1998**, *123*, 93–97. [CrossRef]

124. Iranpour, R.; Zandian, A.; Mohammadizadeh, M.; Mohammadzadeh, A.; Balali-Mood, M.; Hajiheydari, M. Comparison of maternal and umbilical cord blood selenium levels in term and preterm infants. *Chin. J. Contemp. Pediatr.* **2009**, *11*, 513–516.

125. Baxter, I. Ionomics: The functional genomics of elements. *Brief. Funct. Genomics* **2010**, *9*, 149–156. [CrossRef] [PubMed]

126. Zhang, P.; Georgiou, C.A.; Brusic, V. Elemental metabolomics. *Brief. Bioinforma.* **2017**, *19*, 524–536. [CrossRef]

127. Zhang, Y. Trace Elements and Healthcare: A Bioinformatics Perspective. In *Translational Informatics in Smart Healthcare*; Shen, B., Ed.; Springer: Berlin, Germany, 2017; pp. 63–98.

128. Yu, D.; Danku, J.M.; Baxter, I.; Kim, S.; Vatamaniuk, O.K.; Vitek, O.; Ouzzani, M.; Salt, D.E. High-resolution genome-wide scan of genes, gene-networks and cellular systems impacting the yeast ionome. *BMC Genomics* **2012**, *13*, 623. [CrossRef] [PubMed]

129. Huang, X.-Y.; Salt, D.E. Plant ionomics: From elemental profiling to environmental adaptation. *Mol. Plant* **2016**, *9*, 787–797. [CrossRef]

130. Ma, S.; Lee, S.-G.; Kim, E.B.; Park, T.J.; Seluanov, A.; Gorbunova, V.; Buffenstein, R.; Seravalli, J.; Gladyshev, V.N. Organization of the mammalian ionome according to organ origin, lineage specialization, and longevity. *Cell Rep.* **2015**, *13*, 1319–1326. [CrossRef]

131. Malinouski, M.; Hasan, N.M.; Zhang, Y.; Seravalli, J.; Lin, J.; Avanesov, A.; Lutsenko, S.; Gladyshev, V.N. Genome-wide RNAi ionomics screen reveals new genes and regulation of human trace element metabolism. *Nat. Commun.* **2014**, *5*, 3301. [CrossRef] [PubMed]

132. Sun, L.; Yu, Y.; Huang, T.; An, P.; Yu, D.; Yu, Z.; Li, H.; Sheng, H.; Cai, L.; Xue, J. Associations between ionomic profile and metabolic abnormalities in human population. *PLoS ONE* **2012**, *7*, e38845. [CrossRef] [PubMed]

133. Herman, M.; Golasik, M.; Piekoszewski, W.; Walas, S.; Napierala, M.; Wyganowska-Swiatkowska, M.; Kurhanska-Flisykowska, A.; Wozniak, A.; Florek, E. Essential and Toxic Metals in Oral Fluid–a Potential Role in the Diagnosis of Periodontal Diseases. *Biol. Trace Elem. Res.* **2016**, *173*, 275–282. [CrossRef] [PubMed]

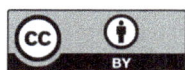

![nutrients logo] *nutrients*

MDPI

Article

Factors Associated with Serum 25-Hydroxyvitamin D Concentration in Two Cohorts of Pregnant Women in Southern Ontario, Canada

Maude Perreault [1], Caroline J. Moore [1], Gerhard Fusch [1], Koon K. Teo [2] and Stephanie A. Atkinson [1,*]

[1]   Department of Pediatrics, McMaster University, Hamilton, L8S 4L8, Canada; perream@mcmaster.ca (M.P.); camoore@mcmaster.ca (C.J.M.); gefusch@mcmaster.ca (G.F.)

[2]   Department of Medicine (Cardiology), McMaster University, Hamilton, L8S 4L8, Canada; teok@mcmaster.ca

*   Correspondence: satkins@mcmaster.ca; Tel.: +1-905-521-2100 (ext. 75644)

Received: 29 November 2018; Accepted: 6 January 2019; Published: 9 January 2019

check for updates

Abstract: Vitamin D deficiency in pregnancy is widely reported, but whether this applies in North America is unclear since no population-based surveys of vitamin D status in pregnancy exist in Canada or the United States. The objectives were to assess (i) the intake and sources of vitamin D, (ii) vitamin D status, and (iii) factors associated with serum 25-hydroxyvitamin D (25-OHD) concentration in two cohorts of pregnant women from Southern Ontario, Canada, studied over a span of 14 years. Maternal characteristics, physical measurements, fasting blood samples and nutrient intake were obtained at enrolment in 332 pregnant women from the Family Atherosclerosis Monitoring In early Life (FAMILY) study and 191 from the Be Healthy in Pregnancy (BHIP) study. Serum 25-OHD was measured by LC/MS-MS. The median (Q1, Q3) total vitamin D intake was 383 IU/day (327, 551) in the FAMILY study and 554 IU/day (437, 796) in the BHIP study. Supplemental vitamin D represented 64% of total intake in participants in FAMILY and 78% in BHIP. The mean (SD) serum 25-OHD was 76.5 (32.9) nmol/L in FAMILY and 79.7 (22.3) nmol/L in BHIP. Being of European descent and blood sampling in the summer season were significantly associated with a higher maternal serum 25-OHD concentration. In summary, health care practitioners should be aware that vitamin D status is sufficient in the majority of pregnant Canadian women of European ancestry, likely due to sun exposure.

Keywords: serum 25-OHD; pregnancy; developmental origins of health and disease; bone health

---

1. Introduction

Adequate maternal vitamin D status is critical to pregnancy health outcomes and the vitamin D status of the infant at birth, and may program for bone development in childhood and later life [1–3]. Vitamin D is essential for bone mineralization, proper bone accretion and growth of the fetus during pregnancy [4]. Systematic reviews of randomized studies identified the effects of maternal vitamin D supplementation on reducing low birth weight prevalence and improving infant growth, with some indications of its potential benefit on pregnancy complications such as pre-eclampsia [5–7]. Maternal vitamin D status in pregnancy has also been positively associated with bone health outcomes in infants [8], children [9,10] and adolescents [11].

Given the potential health benefits of vitamin D, supplementation has gained popularity in the general public over the last decade. The dose in common brands of prenatal multivitamins in Canada has increased from 300 to 600 IU/pill on average over the years, but doses of over-the-counter multi-nutrient supplements range from 200 to 1000 IU/tablet, and single vitamin D supplements are available in doses of 1000–10,000 IU/tablet. As well, the consumption of vitamin D fortified products is gaining popularity in the market as pregnant women become aware of the possible benefits of vitamin D during and after pregnancy.

Despite the potential importance of maternal vitamin D status on the health outcomes of mother and child, no population-based data exist as pregnant women have not been sampled in the nutrition and health surveys in Canada or the United States to date. Claims of a "pandemic" or a high prevalence of vitamin D deficiency in pregnant and lactating women in Canada [12] are not founded on population-based surveys, but rather, cite literature primarily from Afro-American and Indigenous groups living in Canada. In a single US study [13], it was postulated that intakes of 4000 IU of vitamin D per day during pregnancy are required to optimize the production of 1,25-dihydroxyvitamin D (1,25-OH$_2$D) and cord blood 25-hydroxyvitamin D (25-OHD). However, no study to date has demonstrated that vitamin D intakes in pregnancy of >400 up to 4000 IU/day result in any functional benefits to mother or infant. Thus, in the recently revised Dietary Reference Intakes (DRI) [14], the Estimated Average Requirement (EAR) for vitamin D in pregnancy is the same as for non-pregnant women at 400 IU per day. This recommendation was confirmed by the Scientific Advisory Committee on Nutrition in the United Kingdom [15], as well as by the European Food Safety Authority in Europe [16].

The present study was undertaken with the objective to assess (i) the intake and sources of vitamin D, (ii) the vitamin D status, and (iii) the factors associated with maternal serum 25-OHD concentration as a measure of vitamin D status in two cohorts of pregnant women living in Southern Ontario, Canada, studied over a span of 14 years.

2. Materials and Methods

2.1. Study Design

Pregnant women enrolled in the FAMILY and BHIP studies were included, both of which were conducted in accordance with the Declaration of Helsinki. The Family Atherosclerosis Monitoring In early Life (FAMILY) study was a longitudinal, prospective birth cohort study designed to investigate the determinants of obesity, type 2 diabetes and cardiometabolic traits early in life [17]. A total of 857 pregnant women were recruited through three hospitals in Hamilton and Burlington, Ontario, Canada between the years of 2002–2009. For this ancillary study on factors associated with maternal serum 25-OHD concentration, separate ethics approval was granted for the assessment of vitamin D status and bone health in subjects of the FAMILY study by the Research Ethics Board at Hamilton Health Sciences/McMaster University (REB #02-060). Participants gave informed written consent for this sub-study. The Be Healthy in Pregnancy (BHIP) Study is an ongoing randomized controlled trial (RCT; Clinical Trials Ref: NCT01693510) [18] for which the primary research objective is to determine whether introducing a structured and monitored nutrition and exercise program in early pregnancy, compared to standard prenatal care, will increase the number of women attaining gestational weight gain within the Institute of Medicine (IOM), Health and Medicine Division recommendations for their pre-pregnancy body mass index (BMI) category [19]. The present analysis included data obtained at baseline prior to randomization. Between the years 2012–2018, 274 healthy pregnant women were recruited from health care clinics in Hamilton, Burlington and London, Ontario. Informed written consent was obtained upon study enrolment. Ethics approval was obtained from the Research Ethics Boards of Hamilton Health Sciences (REB Project#12-469), Western Ontario in London (HSREB 103272), and Joseph Brant Hospital in Burlington (JBH 000-018-14), all in Southern Ontario, Canada.

2.2. Maternal Data Collection

Maternal demographics, pregnancy history, fasting blood samples and physical measurements were obtained from each participant upon study entry. For the FAMILY study, the information and blood samples were obtained between 24 and 36 weeks of gestation, while for the BHIP study, they were collected between 12 and 17 weeks of gestation. Maternal height and weight were measured, gestational weight gain was self-reported and pre-pregnancy BMI was calculated. Ethnicity, education level and annual household income were self-reported. Maternal health behaviours were self-reported using questionnaires. For the FAMILY study, participants completed a validated semi-quantitative multi-ethnic food frequency questionnaire (FFQ) including supplements [20,21] Nutrient composition was calculated as previously described [22], excluding records where the FFQ was <50% incomplete, or with implausible dietary intakes (<500 or >4500 kcal/day). For the BHIP study, participants completed diet records for three consecutive days (two weekdays and one weekend day) including both foods and supplements, as used previously in pregnant women [23]. Participants were asked to weigh the foods eaten when possible, using household measures such as cups/spoons when weight was not able to be determined. No diet records with implausible intakes were found in the BHIP study. Diet records were analyzed using Nutritionist Pro diet analysis software (Version 5.2, Axxya Systems, Stafford, TX, USA), and the Canadian Nutrient File (version 2015) to obtain daily intake of vitamin D. For the FAMILY study, dairy products were classified as low fat ($\leq$2% fat) or regular fat ($\geq$3.25% fat) dairy products. For the BHIP study, the categories were milk (low and regular fat combined), yogurt (low and regular fat combined), and other dairy products (i.e., regular fat sour cream, cream, cheese, and ice cream). In Canada, all milk and margarine products are fortified with vitamin D_3 by law. Yogurt and other dairy products are sometimes made from vitamin D_3 fortified milk, and this is noted on the label. Exercise was self-reported by participants in both studies. In the FAMILY study, participants completed a validated questionnaire [24], and were categorized as currently exercising or not. In the BHIP study, participants reported exercising or not at recruitment by completing the Physical Activity Readiness Medical Examination (PARmed-X) for Pregnancy [25].

2.3. Vitamin D Analysis

Serum 25-OHD (D_2 and D_3 isomers) was measured by ultra-performance liquid chromatography tandem mass spectrometry (UPLC-MS/MS) using the Waters application note 720002748 [26] with a modified sample preparation that included a saponification step [27]. Saponification prevents fat droplet formation in the supernatant after extraction, which can occur in plasma with a high triglyceride concentration. Saponification converts triacylglycerides into water-soluble fatty acid soaps. This is particularly important as circulating lipids can be elevated in pregnant women [28]. In short, 150 µL of serum and 10 µL of internal standard solution (800 nmol/L, 25-OHD$_3$-d$_6$; 99% pure; Medical Isotopes, Pelham, NH, USA) were vortexed and 50 µL of methanol (Fisher Scientific, Ottawa, Ontario, Canada), 100 µL of ascorbic acid (20% w/v, (>99.9% pure); Sigma Aldrich, Oakville, Canada) and 40 µL of potassium hydroxide (45% w/v; Fluka Analytical, Ronkonkoma, NY, USA) were added. Samples were placed in a 75 °C hot water bath for 20 minutes. After cooling down to room temperature, the mixture was extracted with 500 µL of heptane (Fluka Analytical, Ronkonkoma, NY, USA). The organic phase was evaporated under a gentle stream of nitrogen, and reconstituted in 75 µL of methanol (MS grade, Fisher Scientific, Ottawa, Ontario, Canada). The accuracy and precision of the LC-MS/MS method for measuring 25-OHD$_2$ and 25-OHD$_3$ was evaluated using National Institute of Standards and Technology (NIST) Standard Reference Material 972a (Bureau of Standards, Washington, DC, USA). 25-OHD$_3$/25-OHD$_2$ serum controls purchased from BioRad (Munich, Germany) served as a daily quality control. A Waters Acquity UPLC/TQD system was used with an Acquity UPLC BEH C18 column. The transitions m/z 401/383 for 25-OHD$_3$, 407/389 for 25-OHD$_3$-d$_6$, and 413.5/395.3 for 25-OHD$_2$ were used for quantification.

2.4. Statistical Analysis

Statistical analysis was performed using JMP®9.0 (Version 9.0.1, SAS Institute Inc., Cary, NC, USA) and GraphPad Prism (Version 7, La Jolla, CA, USA). Descriptive statistics were computed by calculating the means and standard deviations of normally distributed continuous data; medians and quartiles (Q1 and Q3) for non-normally distributed continuous data; and counts and percentages for categorical data. *T*-tests were performed to compare groups and significance was established at $p < 0.05$. Analysis of variance (ANOVA) was performed to compare 25-OHD concentrations in women of different pre-pregnancy BMI categories. Significance was established at $p < 0.05$. Mean values are given as means ± standard deviations if not stated otherwise. To determine which factors were associated with maternal serum 25-OHD concentration, we conducted a multivariable linear regression analysis. The variables of interest included in our multivariable regression were decided a priori based on clinical rationale and evidence from the literature. The non-standardized regression coefficients and their corresponding 95% confidence intervals (CIs) and *p*-values for the multivariable analyses are presented.

3. Results

3.1. Demographics and Physical Characteristics

A total of 332 participants from the FAMILY study and 191 from the BHIP study were included in this report as they had available maternal serum samples analysed for 25-OHD. Participants of the FAMILY study were enrolled at a median of 28 weeks gestation, while the BHIP study participants were enrolled at a median of 13 weeks gestation. Half of the FAMILY participants (54%) were enrolled by 2006 and all by 2009, while most participants (96%) of the BHIP study were enrolled between 2013 and 2017. The mean (SD) age of the participants was significantly higher in the FAMILY study than in the BHIP study (32.5 (4.7) vs. 31.2 (3.9) years; $p = 0.001$). Pre-pregnancy BMI was not statistically different between studies (Table 1). According to the pre-pregnancy BMI data, about half of the participants had normal weight, while half were categorized as overweight or obese upon entering pregnancy (Table 1). Most participants were of European ancestry, had a tertiary level of education, and were currently exercising. Few participants in the FAMILY study and none in the BHIP smoked during pregnancy, the latter because it was an exclusion criterion.

Table 1. Demographic, lifestyle and physical characteristics of participants during pregnancy.

Maternal Characteristics	FAMILY Study N = 332		BHIP Study N = 191	
	N	(%)	N	(%)
Gestational age	24–36 weeks		12–17 weeks	
Pre-pregnancy BMI (kg/m^2)				
Underweight (<18.5)	4	1	3	1
Normal weight (18.5–24.9)	144	45	91	48
Overweight (25.0–29.9)	103	32	61	32
Obese (≥30)	69	22	36	19
Unknown	12	-	0	-
Ethnicity				
European descent	285	86	171	90
Other	47	14	20	10
Household income (CAD)				
<$50,000	68	21	15	8
$50,000–$99,999	138	43	91	48
≥$100,000	111	35	79	41
Unknown	15	1	6	3
Education (years)				
≤13	46	14	0	0
>13	286	86	191	100
Smoking status				
Smoked during pregnancy	10	3	0	0
Former smoker; quit before pregnancy	107	33	n/a	n/a
Never smoked	212	64	n/a	n/a
Unknown	3	-	n/a	n/a

Table 1. *Cont.*

	FAMILY Study $N = 332$		**BHIP Study** $N = 191$	
Maternal Characteristics	N	(%)	N	(%)
Gestational age	24–36 weeks		12–17 weeks	
Exercise at study entry				
Not currently exercising	49	15	42	22
Currently exercising	283	85	147	77
Missing data	0	-	2	1

Data not applicable (n/a) as smoking status was an exclusion criteria in the BHIP study, and such data was not collected.

3.2. Intake of Vitamin D in Both Studies: Trend Over 10 Years

The median (Q1, Q3) total vitamin D intake in the FAMILY study was 383 IU/day (327, 551) with the highest intake being 3050 IU/day (Figure 1). The median total vitamin D intake in the BHIP Study was 554 IU/day (437, 796) with the highest intake being 11,062 IU/day. Intakes of vitamin D met the EAR of 400 IU/day in 43% of participants in the FAMILY study and 80% in the BHIP study. Vitamin intake from food sources alone met the EAR in only 9% of participants in both the FAMILY and BHIP studies (Figure 1). No participants in the FAMILY study exceeded the Tolerable Upper Intake Level (UL) of 4000 IU/day, and only three participants in the BHIP (2%) exceeded the UL. Supplement intake represented 64% (289 IU/day) of total intake in the FAMILY study and 78% (629 IU/day) in the BHIP study. Supplements containing vitamin D, mostly prenatal multivitamins, were consumed by 87% of participants in the FAMILY study. The median (Q1, Q3) intake of vitamin D from multivitamins was 300 IU/day (300, 300) but ranged from 0 to 3000 IU/day. In the BHIP study, 92% of participants were consuming supplements containing vitamin D. The median (Q1, Q3) intake of vitamin D from multivitamins was 400 IU/day (400, 600), ranging from 0 to 11,000 IU/day for some participants.

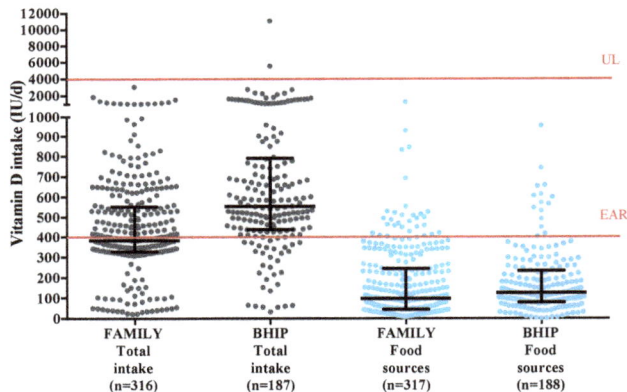

Figure 1. Maternal dietary intake of vitamin D of participants in the FAMILY and BHIP studies. Median and interquartile ranges are displayed for total intake and food sources contribution to total vitamin D. — Vitamin D recommendations for pregnancy: Estimated Average Requirement (EAR) = 400 IU/day; Tolerable Upper Intake Level (UL) = 4000 IU/day [14].

3.3. Maternal Serum 25-OHD Concentration during Pregnancy

The mean serum 25-OHD concentration was in the optimal range (serum 25-OHD 50–125 nmol/L [14]). The isomer 25-OHD$_2$ was detected in only 6% of participants in the BHIP study (data not available for the FAMILY study) at a concentration of 0.51 ± 2.89 nmol/L (mean ± SD); thus, the D2 isomer did not contribute significantly to the overall total serum 25-OHD. Accordingly, the total circulating 25-OHD is a reflection of 25-OHD$_3$. Serum 25-OHD concentrations did not differ between women with different pre-pregnancy BMI values in either study (Table 2). The season that blood was drawn was significantly associated with 25-OHD concentrations in both studies, where blood samples collected in summer had higher serum 25-OHD than in winter (p = 0.001 in FAMILY and p = 0.002 in BHIP). The threshold representing a sufficient 25-OHD concentration of 50 nmol/L as set by the IOM [14] was met or exceeded by 77% of participants in the FAMILY study and 93% of participants in the BHIP study (Figure 2). The range of maternal 25-OHD concentrations was greater in the FAMILY study compared to in the BHIP study; 5% of participants in the FAMILY study had serum 25-OHD in the deficient range (<30 nmol/L) and 9% of participants exceeded 125 nmol/L, the level for excessive circulating 25-OHD. In the BHIP study, only 0.5% of participants were clinically deficient, while 3% surpassed the excessive threshold. No correlation was observed in the FAMILY study between maternal total vitamin D intake and maternal serum 25-OHD concentration (R^2 = 0.01, p = 0.09). In the BHIP study, a higher total intake of vitamin D was associated with higher serum 25-OHD (R^2 = 0.11, p < 0.0001). For BHIP, supplements contributed an important amount to the total vitamin D intake and contributed to a higher 25-OHD concentration (Figure 3).

Table 2. Maternal serum 25-OHD concentration by season of blood draw and pre-pregnancy body mass index (BMI) category.

Category	FAMILY Study			BHIP Study		
	Serum 25-OHD, nmol/L Mean (SD) (95% CI)	N (%)	*p*-value	Serum 25-OHD, nmol/L Mean (SD) (95% CI)	N (%)	*p*-value
All participants	76.5 (32.9) (72.9, 80.1)	332	-	79.7 (22.3) (76.5, 82.9)	191	-
Season of blood draw						
Summer (May–Oct.)	83.47 (34.3) (78.3, 88.7)	169 (51)	0.0001	84.9 (21.0) (80.9, 89.0)	106 (55)	0.0002
Winter (Nov–Apr.)	68.5 (29.3) (63.9, 73.1)	160 (48)		73.2 (22.2) (68.4, 78.0)	85 (45)	
Missing data	-	3 (1)		-	-	
Pre-pregnancy BMI (kg/m^2)						
Underweight (<18.5)	72.2 (44.3) (1.6, 142.8)	4 (1)		90.3 (15.1) (52.6, 127.9)	3 (1)	
Normal (18.5–24.9)	79.5 (33.4) (74.0, 85.0)	144 (43)	0.11	82.2 (21.2) (77.8, 86.5)	93 (49)	0.10
Overweight (25.0–29.9)	78.3 (33.7) (71.7, 84.9)	103 (31)		73.8 (20.5) (68.4, 79.2)	58 (31)	
Obese (≥30)	68.1 (30.0) (60.9, 75.3)	69 (21)		81.8 (26.6) (90.7, 73,0)	37 (19)	
Missing data	-	12 (4)		-	-	

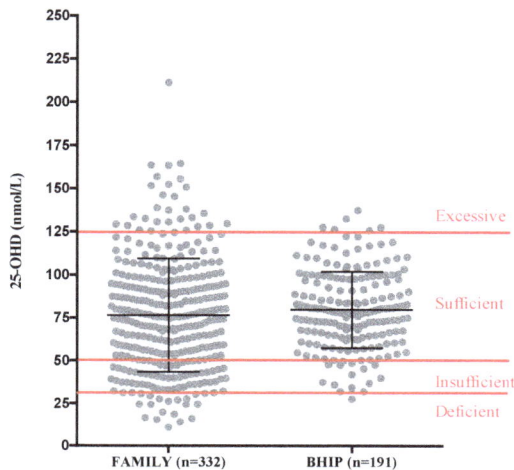

Figure 2. Maternal serum 25-OHD concentration (mean, SD) in participants from the FAMILY and BHIP studies in comparison to the recommendations by the Institute of Medicine [14]; — <30 nmol/L deficient, 30–50 nmol/L insufficient, ≥50 nmol/L sufficient, >125 nmol/L excessive.

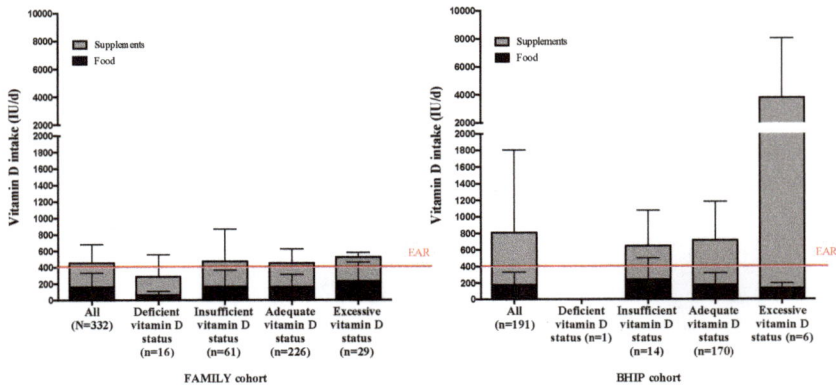

Figure 3. Total vitamin D intake in the FAMILY and BHIP studies, by maternal serum 25-OHD concentration. Mean and standard deviation are displayed. The Estimated Average Requirement (EAR) is indicated by — [14].

3.4. Factors Associated with Maternal Serum 25-OHD Concentrations in Pregnancy

For participants enrolled in the FAMILY study, a multivariable analysis demonstrated that a higher maternal 25-OHD concentration was significantly associated with being of European descent, having blood drawn in summer, and having a low pre-pregnancy BMI (Table 3).

For participants enrolled in the BHIP study, a multivariable analysis revealed that higher maternal 25-OHD concentrations were significantly associated with having blood drawn in summer and vitamin D intake from regular fat dairy products (i.e., sour cream, cream, ice cream, cheese) (Table 3).

Table 3. Multivariable analysis of factors associated with maternal serum 25-OHD concentrations during pregnancy in the FAMILY and BHIP studies.

Variables	FAMILY Study			BHIP Study		
	Estimated Coefficient	95% CI	*p*-Value	Estimated Coefficient	95% CI	*p*-Value
Ethnicity (European descent as reference)	−5.85	−10.97, −0.72	**0.025**	−5.91	−12.44, 0.61	0.075
Season of blood draw for baseline blood (Winter as reference)	**7.73**	**4.27, 11.18**	**<0.001**	**8.27**	**4.44, 12.09**	**<0.001**
Exercising at enrollment	0.53	−5.73, 4.66	0.840	3.08	−1.72, 7.88	0.206
Pre-pregnancy BMI	−0.92	**−1.52, −0.31**	**0.003**	−0.37	−1.19, 0.46	0.381
Total vitamin D intake	−0.01	−0.04, 0.02	0.469	−0.01	−0.04, 0.02	0.451
Vitamin D intake from supplement	0.01	−0.02, 0.05	0.422	0.02	−0.01, 0.05	0.174
Vitamin D intake from milk	1.03	−3.97, 6.02	0.687	0.03	−0.03, 0.10	0.272
Vitamin D intake from low fat dairy products	4.19	−0.43, 8.82	0.076	-	-	-
Vitamin D intake from regular fat dairy products (sour cream, cream, ice cream, cheese)	−2.11	−5.99, 1.77	0.285	**0.44**	**0.08, 0.81**	**0.017**

Bold format for significant results.

4. Discussion

The majority of healthy pregnant women in Southern Ontario in the last 10 years have had sufficient circulating 25-OHD both in early and late pregnancy using the reference cut-off values from the DRI report [14]. While risk for vitamin D deficiency may exist globally [29], this does not appear to apply to pregnant women living in Southern Ontario. Health care practitioners should be aware that in our community, <5% of pregnant women had serum 25-OHD <30 nmol/L, which is similar to what was found in the general Canadian population (4%, defined as <27.5 nmol/L) by the Canadian Health Measures Survey (CHMS) [30]. The overall circulating 25-OHD in the participants in the two combined pregnant cohorts was 77.7 nmol/L, a value slightly higher than the average serum 25-OHD of 69.5 nmol/L reported for females of child-bearing age (20–39 years old) in the CHMS [30], and which is significantly higher than observed in males in the same age category. The latter is likely attributable to higher vitamin supplement intake among females [30]. High intakes of supplements containing vitamin D were observed in our two cohorts of pregnant women where approximately 90% were taking prenatal supplements. Vitamin D supplementation is known to be associated with higher 25-OHD status, but the response can be highly heterogeneous among pregnant women [7,31], including those in our study. Despite the majority of participants taking prenatal supplements in both the FAMILY and BHIP studies, heterogeneity was indicated, in which prenatal supplement intake was not associated with 25-OHD status in FAMILY ($R^2 = 0.00$, $p = 0.58$) but a modest albeit significant association with 25-OHD status was observed in BHIP ($R^2 = 0.11$, $p < 0.0001$).

Although the average maternal intake of vitamin D from food did not reach the EAR of 400 IU/day and this was only weakly associated with 25-OHD concentration, the estimated total vitamin D intake from both food and supplements exceeded 400 IU/day in only 45% of participants in the FAMILY study but in 80% of the BHIP participants. Our results are in agreement with data reported from Canadian studies showing that the primary source of oral vitamin D (approximately 60% total intake) is supplements [32,33]. In the Canadian food chain, there are limited natural or fortified food sources of vitamin D. According to our data and those of other Canadian studies [32–37], intake of vitamin D supplements is common in pregnancy, and combined with sun exposure, the prevalence of inadequacy of vitamin D intake is low. As noted above, almost all participants in the two cohorts of pregnant women took prenatal supplements (containing between 200 and 600 IU of vitamin D), vitamin D supplements (up to 10,000 IU), or both. Although participants from the BHIP study consumed more vitamin D overall due to higher supplement intake, they had similar 25-OHD concentrations to participants in the FAMILY study. Participants in the FAMILY study presented a broader range of 25-OHD concentrations, likely due to the larger sample size of FAMILY as compared with the BHIP study, with participants at the extremes with either clinical deficiency or excessive 25-OHD concentration. These results also suggest that sun exposure plays an important role through cutaneous production of vitamin D, ensuring most participants achieved an adequate vitamin D status.

The average serum 25-OHD in our participants was moderately higher than that reported since 2000 for Canadian pregnant women in other provinces. In the Vancouver area, pregnant women predominately of European descent ($N = 336$ at 20–35 weeks gestation) had a mean (95% CI) 25-OHD of 66.7 (64.2–69.1) nmol/L [34]. In a larger study in Québec City and Halifax ($N = 1635$ at 12–15 weeks gestation, primarily of European descent), the mean (SD) 25-OHD was 52.7 (16.9) nmol/L [38]. Further, in Edmonton and Calgary, Alberta ($N = 537$, primarily of European ancestry), the mean (SD) serum 25-OHD was 93.3 (25.6) nmol/L in the first trimester and 95.3 (25) nmol/L in the second trimester of pregnancy [36]. The 25-OHD concentration of women in our study is comparable to the first two studies but lower than reported by the APrON study in Alberta [36]. These discrepancies in 25-OHD concentration may be due to participants' exposure to sun, the nature of the study samples, where multiethnic participants have lower 25-OHD concentration [34], and because those with the highest socioeconomic status have the highest 25-OHD concentration [36]. In addition, the largest consumers of multivitamin supplements are found in Alberta, while the lowest consumers are in Quebec [30]. Discrepancies can also result from the methods used to measure serum 25-OHD—either by ELISA [34,38] or LC-MS/MS [36]. In all cohorts, the prevalence of deficiency was very low (either defined as 25-OHD < 25 nmol/L [38] or < 30 nmol/L [34,36]); from < 1 to 7% [34,36,38], aligning with our observed prevalence deficiency (defined as 25-OHD < 30 nmol/L) of 5% in FAMILY and <1% BHIP studies. The prevalence of insufficient 25-OHD (< 50 nmol/L) in these cohorts was between 2% and 45% [34,36,38], similar to what we observed in the FAMILY study (18%) and BHIP study (7%).

Based on the contemporary studies noted above and using the IOM reference values, the majority of Canadian women have an adequate serum 25-OHD concentration in pregnancy, regardless of stage of pregnancy. However, controversy remains as to the 'optimal' 25-OHD concentration in pregnancy, since the clinical significance both for mother and infant of a 25-OHD above 50 nmol/L is still undefined [7,39–41]. Data from a recent systematic review suggests that pregnant women with bacterial vaginosis, gestational diabetes, pre-eclampsia and those with small for gestational age (SGA) babies have lower circulating 25-OHD than their healthy pregnant counterparts [42,43]. However, the value for what constitutes 'lower 25-OHD' was not defined in the review and their analysis included individual studies that used both 50 and 75 nmol/L as the cut-off for sufficiency. Conversely, a further systematic review of randomized controlled trials found no clear evidence for maternal benefits or reduced incidence of pre-term birth with supplementation of 25-OHD. In this review, only eight out of 43 trials were categorized as having an overall low risk of bias [39]. Many of the trials included in this review were small and of low quality; therefore, more research is needed before recommendations on optimal vitamin D status in pregnancy can be made. Further, a large prospective cohort study from New Zealand found that serum 25-OHD concentrations in pregnant women were not associated with pre-eclampsia, SGA babies or pre-term birth; however, of note, this population was largely 25-OHD replete [44].

Controversy also exists as to the optimal target for serum 25-OHD in pregnancy. A higher maternal 25-OHD concentration at delivery has been associated with infant cord blood 25-OHD status, and maternal use of vitamin D supplements was associated with higher odds of reaching sufficiency (defined as >75 nmol/L) for both mothers and infants [45]. However, uncertainty exists as to whether a higher maternal 25-OHD concentration (i.e., 25-OHD > 75 nmol/L) in pregnancy is linked with health benefits. It has been hypothesized that the optimal 25-OHD concentration would be the one leading to maximal conversion to the active form of vitamin D [46]. To that effect, data from one recent randomized trial were interpreted to indicate the total circulating 25-OHD must reach 100 nmol/L in order to optimize circulating $1,25-OH_2D$ in pregnancy [47]. In that case, only 21% of participants in our cohort would have met or exceeded this 25-OHD concentration. In contrast to benefits, high maternal, cord and infant 25-OHD concentrations may have disadvantageous effects on infant growth. In an RCT including 798 mother and infant dyads, mothers with pregnancy 25-OHD > 125 nmol/L had the smallest infants at 6 months [48]. Further, an evidence-based consensus statement determined that there is little evidence for any benefits of maternal vitamin D supplementation on early life anthropometry and growth in the offspring or on clinical benefits for the mother [49]. It was concluded that the cut-off for vitamin D sufficient status of 50 nmol/L, as suggested by the DRI, remains the accepted standard [49]. Based on our data, with the current level of vitamin D fortification in Canada the use of supplements might be essential for pregnant women to reach the EAR for vitamin D, but is not the most important factor in ensuring participants have adequate vitamin D status. Summer season, and by inference, amount of sun exposure, appeared to have the strongest impact on maternal serum 25-OHD concentration in our cohorts.

The factors that were significantly associated with maternal 25-OHD concentrations in this study are in agreement with reported maternal factors in pregnant women across Canada (Vancouver, Halifax and Québec City, Edmonton and Calgary). Summer season at time of blood draw [34,38] and being of European ancestry [34] were reported as significant factors associated with 25-OHD concentration in Canadian pregnant women living in Southern Ontario. While a pre-pregnancy BMI < 25 kg/m^2 was associated with a higher maternal 25-OHD concentration compared to pre-pregnancy BMI ≥ 35 kg/m^2 [38]; a relationship between pre-pregnancy BMI and maternal 25-OHD was observed in the FAMILY study but not in the BHIP study. This may relate to the larger sample size in FAMILY. Consumption of milk, a mandatory vitamin D-fortified food in Canada, was surprisingly not associated with maternal 25-OHD concentrations in either study. Health Canada recently indicated plans to increase the amount of vitamin D for mandatory fortification of milk and margarine in an effort to help Canadians meet the DRIs [50]. Until that comes into effect by the end of 2022, it is likely that milk consumption alone will not be sufficient source of vitamin D intake for Canadian pregnant women.

Our study has several strengths including a detailed dietary intake including food and supplement sources and measurement of serum 25-OHD concentrations by the gold standard LC-MS/MS [51]. The generalizability of the findings may be limited due to the demographic homogeneity (primarily of European descent, highly educated women). Another limitation includes the reporting bias inherent to diet records, but our dietary assessment was combined with direct measurement of nutritional status, providing a better evaluation of nutritional adequacy. Lastly, the lack of quantitative measurement of sun exposure limits the interpretation of the results, as there might be differences between an individual's exposure due to variable time spent in outdoor activities, clothing coverage and use of sunscreen. Future steps include a prospective longitudinal assessment of participants in the BHIP study to investigate the association of maternal 25-OHD concentrations with pregnancy and neonatal health outcomes.

Author Contributions: Conceptualization, S.A.A.; Methodology, S.A.A.; Laboratory work, G.F., C.J.M.; Formal Analysis, M.P., S.A.A.; Investigation, S.A.A., M.P.; Data Curation, M.P., C.J.M., S.A.A.; Writing—Original Draft Preparation, M.P., G.F., S.A.A.; Writing—Review & Editing, M.P., G.F., S.A.A., C.J.M., K.K.T.; Visualization, M.P.; Supervision, S.A.A.; Project Administration, S.A.A.; Funding Acquisition, S.A.A.

Funding: The FAMILY study received separate funding from the Dairy Farmers of Canada to conduct the vitamin D analysis. The core FAMILY study was funded by the Canadian Institutes of Health Research (CIHR) and the Heart and Stroke Foundation. The BHIP study was funded by the CIHR; and the Dairy Cluster by Dairy Farmers of Canada, and Agriculture and Agri-food Canada (AAFC).

Acknowledgments: Authors would like to acknowledge all the families who participated in the FAMILY and BHIP study, as well as the community partners and collaborators involved in these studies. We are grateful for the contributions to data collection by the FAMILY Study team especially Nora Abdalla, and graduate students Melody Ng and Dilisha Rodrigopulle, and the BHIP study team, especially Michelle Mottola, PhD. The statistical consultation by Lehana Thabane, PhD is also gratefully acknowledged.

Conflicts of Interest: The authors declare no conflict of interest. The funders had no role in the design of the study; in the collection, analyses, or interpretation of data; in the writing of the manuscript, or in the decision to publish the results.

References

1. Heyden, E.L.; Wimalawansa, S.J. Vitamin D: Effects on human reproduction, pregnancy, and fetal well-being. *J. Steroid Biochem. Mol. Biol.* **2017**, *180*, 41–50. [CrossRef] [PubMed]
2. Larqué, E.; Morales, E.; Leis, R.; Blanco-Carnero, J.E. Maternal and foetal health implications of vitamin D status during pregnancy. *Ann. Nutr. Metab.* **2018**, *72*, 179–192. [CrossRef] [PubMed]
3. Curtis, E.M.; Moon, R.J.; Harvey, N.C.; Cooper, C. Maternal vitamin D supplementation during pregnancy. *Br. Med. Bull.* **2018**, *126*, 57–77. [CrossRef] [PubMed]
4. Kovacs, C.S. Calcium, phosphorus, and bone metabolism in the fetus and newborn. *Early Hum. Dev.* **2015**, *11*, 6–11. [CrossRef] [PubMed]
5. Thorne-Lyman, A.; Fawzi, W.W. Vitamin D during pregnancy and maternal, neonatal and infant health outcomes: A systematic review and meta-analysis. *Paediatr. Perinat. Epidemiol.* **2012**, *26*, 75–90. [CrossRef] [PubMed]
6. Bi, W.G.; Nuyt, A.M.; Weiler, H.; Leduc, L.; Santamaria, C.; Wei, S.Q. Association between vitamin D supplementation during pregnancy and offspring growth, morbidity, and mortality. *JAMA Pediatr.* **2018**, *172*, 635–645. [CrossRef] [PubMed]
7. De-Regil, L.; Palacios, C.; Lombardo, L.; Peña-Rosas, J. Vitamin D supplementation for women during pregnancy. *Cochrane Database Syst. Rev.* **2016**. [CrossRef]

8. Viljakainen, H.T.; Saarnio, E.; Hytinantti, T.; Miettinen, M.; Surcel, H.; Mäkitie, O.; Andersson, S.; Laitinen, K.; Lamberg-Allardt, C. Maternal vitamin D status determines bone variables in the newborn. *J. Clin. Endocrinol. Metab.* **2010**, *95*, 1749–1757. [CrossRef]

9. Javaid, M.K.; Crozier, S.R.; Harvey, N.C.; Gale, C.R.; Dennison, E.M.; Boucher, B.J.; Arden, N.K.; Godfrey, K.M.; Cooper, C.; Princess Anne Hospital Study, G. Maternal vitamin D status during pregnancy and childhood bone mass at age 9 years: A longitudinal study. *Lancet* **2006**, *367*, 36–43. [CrossRef]

10. Viljakainen, H.T.; Korhonen, T.; Hytinantti, T.; Laitinen, E.K.A.; Andersson, S.; Mäkitie, O.; Lamberg-Allardt, C. Maternal vitamin D status affects bone growth in early childhood—A prospective cohort study. *Osteoporos. Int.* **2011**, *22*, 883–891. [CrossRef]

11. Zhu, K.; Whitehouse, A.J.; Hart, P.H.; Kusel, M.; Mountain, J.; Lye, S.; Pennell, C.; Walsh, J.P. Maternal vitamin D status during pregnancy and bone mass in offspring at 20 years of age: A prospective cohort study. *J. Bone Min. Res.* **2014**, *29*, 1088–1095. [CrossRef] [PubMed]

12. Godel, J.C.; Canadian Paediatric Society; First Nations, Inuit and Métis Health Committee. Vitamin D supplementation: Recommendations for Canadian mothers and infants. *Paediatr. Child Health* **2007**, *12*, 583–589. [CrossRef]

13. Hollis, B.W. Vitamin D supplementation during pregnancy: Double-blind, randomized clinical trial of safety and effectiveness. *J. Bone Miner. Res.* **2011**, *26*, 2341–2357. [CrossRef] [PubMed]

14. Ross, A.; Taylor, C.; Yaktine, A. *Dietary Reference Intakes for Vitamin D and Calcium*; National Academies Press: Washington, DC, USA, 2011.

15. Scientific Advisory Committee on Nutrition. *Vitamin D and Health*; Assets Publishing Service: London, UK, 2016.

16. EFSA Panel on Dietetic Products Nutrition values for vitamin D. *EFSA J.* **2016**, *14*, e04547. [CrossRef]

17. Morrison, K.M.; Atkinson, S.A.; Yusuf, S.; Bourgeois, J.; McDonald, S.; McQueen, M.J.; Persadie, R.; Hunter, B.; Pogue, J.; Teo, K. The Family Atherosclerosis Monitoring In earLY life (FAMILY) study. Rationale, design, and baseline data of a study examining the early determinants of atherosclerosis. *Am. Heart J.* **2009**, *158*, 533–539. [CrossRef] [PubMed]

18. Perreault, M.; Atkinson, S.A.; Mottola, M.F.; Phillips, S.M.; Bracken, K.; Hutton, E.K.; Xie, F.; Meyre, D.; Morassut, R.E.; Prapavessis, H.; et al. Structured diet and exercise guidance in pregnancy to improve health in women and their offspring: Study protocol for the Be Healthy in Pregnancy (BHIP) randomized controlled trial. *Trials* **2018**, *19*, 691. [CrossRef] [PubMed]

19. Health Canada Prenatal Nutrition Guidelines for Health Professionals, Gestational Weight Gain. Available online: http://www.hc-sc.gc.ca/fn-an/alt_formats/pdf/nutrition/prenatal/ewba-mbsa-eng.pdf2010 (accessed on 24 January 2013).

20. Anand, S.S.; Yusuf, S.; Vuksan, V.; Devanesen, S.; Montague, P.; Kelemen, L.; Bosch, J.; Sigouin, C.; Teo, K.K.; Lonn, E.; et al. The Study of Health Assessment and Risk in Ethnic groups (SHARE): Rationale and design. The SHARE Investigators. *Can. J. Cardiol.* **1998**, *14*, 1349–1357.

21. Kelemen, L.E.; Anand, S.S.; Vuksan, V.; Yi, Q.; Teo, K.K.; Devanesen, S.; Yusuf, S.; Investigators, S. Development and evaluation of cultural food frequency questionnaires for South Asians, Chinese, and Europeans in North America. *J. Am. Diet. Assoc.* **2003**, *103*, 1178–1184. [CrossRef]

22. Merchant, A.T.; Kelemen, L.E.; De Koning, L.; Lonn, E.; Vuksan, V.; Jacobs, R.; Davis, B.; Teo, K.K.; Yusuf, S.; Anand, S.S. Interrelation of saturated fat, trans fat, alcohol intake, and subclinical atherosclerosis. *Am. J. Clin. Nutr.* **2008**, *87*, 168–174. [CrossRef]

23. Mottola, M.F.; Giroux, I.; Gratton, R.; Hammond, J.A.; Hanley, A.; Harris, S.; McManus, R.; Davenport, M.H.; Sopper, M.M. Nutrition and exercise prevent excess weight gain in overweight pregnant women. *Med. Sci. Sport. Exerc.* **2010**, *42*, 265–272. [CrossRef] [PubMed]

24. Held, C.; Iqbal, R.; Lear, S.A.; Rosengren, A.; Islam, S.; Mathew, J.; Yusuf, S. Physical activity levels, ownership of goods promoting sedentary behaviour and risk of myocardial infarction: Results of the INTERHEART study. *Eur. Heart J.* **2012**, *33*, 452–466. [CrossRef] [PubMed]

25. Davies, G.; Wolfe, L.; Mottola, M.; MacKinnon, C. Joint SOGC/CSEP clinical practice guideline: Exercise in pregnancy and the postpartum period. *Can. J. Appl. Physiol.* **2003**, *28*, 330–341. [CrossRef] [PubMed]

26. The Analysis of 25-Hydroxyvitamin D in Serum Using UPLC/MS/MS. Available online: http://www.waters.com/webassets/cms/library/docs/720002748_vit_d_application_note.pdf (accessed on 7 January 2019).

27. Hymøller, L.; Jensen, S.K. Vitamin D analysis in plasma by high performance liquid chromatography (HPLC) with C30 reversed phase column and UV detection—Easy and acetonitrile-free. *J. Chromatogr. A* **2011**, *1218*, 1835–1841. [CrossRef] [PubMed]

28. Perichart-Perera, O.; Muñoz-Manrique, C.; Reyes-López, A.; Tolentino-Dolores, M.; Espino Y Sosa, S.; Ramírez-González, M.C. Metabolic markers during pregnancy and their association with maternal and newborn weight status. *PLoS ONE* **2017**, *12*, e0180874. [CrossRef] [PubMed]

29. Roth, D.E.; Abrams, S.A.; Aloia, J.; Bergeron, G.; Bourassa, M.W.; Brown, K.H.; Calvo, M.S.; Cashman, K.D.; Combs, G.; De-Regil, L.M.; et al. Global prevalence and disease burden of vitamin D deficiency: A roadmap for action in low- and middle-income countries. *Ann. N. Y. Acad. Sci.* **2018**, 1–36. [CrossRef] [PubMed]

30. Langlois, K.; Greene-Finestone, L.; Little, J.; Hidiroglou, N.; Whiting, S. Vitamin D status of Canadians as measured in the 2007 to 2009 Canadian Health Measures Survey. *Stat. Can.* **2010**, *21*, 47–55.

31. Moon, R.J.; Harvey, N.C.; Cooper, C.; D 'angelo, S.; Crozier, S.R.; Inskip, H.M.; Schoenmakers, I.; Prentice, A.; Arden, N.K.; Bishop, N.J.; et al. Determinants of the maternal 25-hydroxyvitamin D response to vitamin D supplementation during pregnancy. *J. Clin. Endocrinol. Metab.* **2016**, *101*, 5012–5020. [CrossRef]

32. Morisset, A.-S.; Weiler, H.A.; Dubois, L.; Ashley-Martin, J.; Shapiro, G.D.; Dodds, L.; Massarelli, I.; Vigneault, M.; Arbuckle, T.E.; Fraser, W.D. Rankings of iron, vitamin D, and calcium intakes in relation to maternal characteristics of pregnant Canadian women. *Appl. Physiol. Nutr. Metab.* **2016**, *41*, 749–757. [CrossRef]

33. Dubois, L.; Diasparra, M.; Bédard, B.; Colapinto, C.K.; Fontaine-Bisson, B.; Tremblay, R.E.; Fraser, W.D. Adequacy of nutritional intake during pregnancy in relation to prepregnancy BMI: Results from the 3D Cohort Study. *Br. J. Nutr.* **2018**, *120*, 335–344. [CrossRef]

34. Li, W.; Green, T.J.; Innis, S.M.; Barr, S.I.; Whiting, S.J.; Shand, A.; von Dadelszen, P. Suboptimal vitamin D levels in pregnant women despite supplement use. *Can. J. Public Health* **2011**, *102*, 308–312.

35. Gomez, M.F.; Field, C.J.; Olstad, D.L.; Loehr, S.; Ramage, S.; Mccargar, L.J.; Kaplan, B.J.; Dewey, D.; Bell, R.C.; Bernier, F.P.; et al. Use of micronutrient supplements among pregnant women in Alberta: Results from the Alberta Pregnancy Outcomes and Nutrition (APrON) cohort. *Matern. Child Nutr.* **2015**, *11*, 497–510. [CrossRef] [PubMed]

36. Aghajafari, F.; Field, C.J.; Kaplan, B.J.; Rabi, D.M.; Maggiore, J.A.; O'Beirne, M.; Hanley, D.A.; Eliasziw, M.; Dewey, D.; Weinberg, A.; et al. The current recommended vitamin D intake guideline for diet and supplements during pregnancy is not adequate to achieve vitamin D sufficiency for most pregnant women. *PLoS ONE* **2016**, *11*, e0157262. [CrossRef] [PubMed]

37. Savard, C.; Lemieux, S.; Weisnagel, S.J.; Fontaine-Bisson, B.; Gagnon, C.; Robitaille, J.; Morisset, A.S. Trimester-specific dietary intakes in a sample of French-Canadian pregnant women in comparison with national nutritional guidelines. *Nutrients* **2018**, *10*, 768. [CrossRef] [PubMed]

38. Woolcott, C.G.; Giguère, Y.; Weiler, H.A.; Spencer, A.; Forest, J.C.; Armson, B.A.; Dodds, L. Determinants of vitamin D status in pregnant women and neonates. *Can. J. Public Health* **2016**, *107*, e410–e416. [CrossRef] [PubMed]

39. Roth, D.E.; Leung, M.; Mesfin, E.; Qamar, H.; Watterworth, J.; Papp, E. Vitamin D supplementation during pregnancy: State of the evidence from a systematic review of randomised trials. *BMJ* **2017**, *359*, j5237. [CrossRef] [PubMed]

40. Eggemoen, Å.R.; Jenum, A.K.; Mdala, I.; Knutsen, K.V.; Lagerlov, P.; Sletner, L. Vitamin D levels during pregnancy and associations with birth weight and body composition of the newborn: A longitudinal multiethnic population-based study. *Br. J. Nutr.* **2017**, *117*, 985–993. [CrossRef] [PubMed]

41. Harvey, N.C.; Holroyd, C.; Ntani, G.; Javaid, K.; Cooper, P.; Moon, R.; Cole, Z.; Tinati, T.; Godfrey, K.; Dennison, E.; et al. Vitamin D supplementation in pregnancy: A systematic review. *Health Technol. Assess.* **2014**, *18*, 1–190. [CrossRef]

42. Aghajafari, F.; Nagulesapillai, T.; Ronksley, P.E.; Tough, S.C.; O'Beirne, M.; Rabi, D.M. Association between maternal serum 25-hydroxyvitamin D level and pregnancy and neonatal outcomes: Systematic review and meta-analysis of observational studies. *BMJ* **2013**, *346*, f1169. [CrossRef]

43. Wei, S.; Qi, H.; Luo, Z.; Fraser, W. Maternal vitamin D status and adverse pregnancy outcomes: A systematic review and meta-analysis. *J. Matern. Neonatal Med.* **2013**, *26*, 889–899. [CrossRef]

44. Boyle, V.T.; Thorstensen, E.B.; Mourath, D.; Jones, M.B.; McCowan, L.M.E.; Kenny, L.C.; Baker, P.N. The relationship between 25-hydroxyvitamin D concentration in early pregnancy and pregnancy outcomes in a large, prospective cohort. *Br. J. Nutr.* **2016**, *116*, 1409–1415. [CrossRef] [PubMed]

45. Aghajafari, F.; Field, C.J.; Kaplan, B.J.; Maggiore, J.A.; O'Beirne, M.; Hanley, D.A.; Eliasziw, M.; Dewey, D.; Ross, S.; Rabi, D. The high prevalence of vitamin D insufficiency in cord blood in Calgary, Alberta (APrON-D Study). *J. Obstet. Gynaecol. Can.* **2017**, *39*, 347–353. [CrossRef] [PubMed]

46. Wagner, C.L.; Hollis, B.W. The Implications of Vitamin D Status During Pregnancy on Mother and her Developing Child. *Front. Endocrinol.* **2018**, *9*, 1–11. [CrossRef] [PubMed]

47. Wagner, C.L.; Taylor, S.N.; Dawodu, A.; Johnson, D.D.; Hollis, B.W. Vitamin D and its role during pregnancy in attaining optimal health of mother and fetus. *Nutrients* **2012**, *4*, 208–230. [CrossRef] [PubMed]

48. Hauta-alus, H.H.; Kajantie, E.; Holmlund-Suila, E.M.; Rosendahl, J.; Valkama, S.M.; Enlund-Cerullo, M.; Helve, O.M.; Hytinantti, T.K.; Viljakainen, H.; Andersson, S.; et al. High pregnancy, cord blood and infant vitamin D concentrations may predict slower infant growth. *J. Clin. Endocrinol. Metab.* **2019**, *104*, 397–407. [CrossRef] [PubMed]

49. Munns, C.F.; Shaw, N.; Kiely, M.; Specker, B.L.; Thacher, T.D.; Ozono, K.; Michigami, T.; Tiosano, D.; Mughal, M.Z.; Makitie, O.; et al. Global consensus recommendations on prevention and management of nutritional rickets. *Horm. Res. Paediatr.* **2016**, *85*, 83–106. [CrossRef] [PubMed]

50. Governement of Canada Summary of Proposed Amendments, Part I: Nutrition Symbols, Other Labelling Provisions, Partially Hydrogenated Oils and Vitamin D. Available online: https://www.canada.ca/en/health-canada/programs/consultation-front-of-package-nutrition-labelling-cgi/summary-of-proposed-amendments.html (accessed on 21 December 2018).

51. Zerwekh, J.E. Blood biomarkers of vitamin D status. *Am. J. Clin. Nutr.* **2008**, *87*, 1087–1091. [CrossRef]

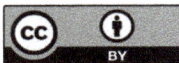

MDPI

St. Alban-Anlage 66

4052 Basel

Switzerland

Tel. +41 61 683 77 34

Fax +41 61 302 89 18

www.mdpi.com

Nutrients Editorial Office

E-mail: nutrients@mdpi.com

www.mdpi.com/journal/nutrients